T0158883

The
Chronic Disease
of
OBESITY

The Chronic Disease

of

OBESITY

How Sponge Syndrome Causes Repeated Weight Gain

Brian Scott Edwards, MD, NFLA

⊙ iUniverse®

THE CHRONIC DISEASE OF OBESITY
HOW SPONGE SYNDROME CAUSES REPEATED WEIGHT GAIN

iUniverse books may be ordered through booksellers or by contacting:

iUniverse
1663 Liberty Drive
Bloomington, IN 47403
www.iuniverse.com
1-800-Authors (1-800-288-4677)

Because of the dynamic nature of the Internet, any web addresses or links contained in this book may have changed since publication and may no longer be valid. The views expressed in this work are solely those of the author and do not necessarily reflect the views of the publisher, and the publisher hereby disclaims any responsibility for them.

Any people depicted in stock imagery provided by Thinkstock are models,
and such images are being used for illustrative purposes only.
Certain stock imagery © Thinkstock.

ISBN: 978-1-5320-4142-6 (sc)
ISBN: 978-1-5320-4143-3 (e)

Library of Congress Control Number: 2018901299

Print information available on the last page.

iUniverse rev. date: 02/01/2018

CONTENTS

Other books written by Brian Scott Edwards MD NFLA

The Fen-Fen Diet Pill Program

The Tubby Theory from Topeka

The Tubby Traveler from Topeka

Dedicated to my wife, Virginia

EPIGRAPH

"The number of fat cells have the last word"
Mark Edwards

FOREWARD

I went to Dr. Brian Edwards as a friend on Oct 22, 2015.

I was desperate as I was not getting better after working with my family physician and two different rheumatologists. My legs were swollen despite being on two diuretics. I was taking allopurinol for the painful bumps on wrists. They finally biopsied the bumps and they consisted of uric acid. My sugar was out of control and I could not lose weight.

Dr. Edwards advised some changes.

I must switch to an Atkins type diet immediately.

Slowly decrease insulin and start slowly increasing invokana.

(On 11-28-15 I was totally off insulin.)

Stop the diuretics.

Start colchicine.

Start metformin up to 2,000 mg a day

Get a sleep apnea test.

Later when the rheumatologist wanted to put me on prednisone, Dr. Edwards said absolutely not to do it and my family physician agreed.

On 1-15-2016 I was on Invokana 300 mg, Metformin 2,000 mg and no insulin my Hgb A1c had dropped from 7.6 to 6.5 with a weight of 318 pounds

Dr Edwards asked my family physician to start Victoza and slowly increase the dose.

On 2-24-16 I was on full Diabetic dose of Victoza 1.8 mg.

My results were miraculous.

Oct 22, 2015
First weigh in at Dr. Edwards home with a Valhalla Total Body Composition scale:
Weight 348 pounds
Body Fat 52.9%
Muscle mass 32.2 pounds
Body Water 38.2%
BMI 57.8

March 8, 2016
I hit a low weight of 308.8
I had lost 40 pounds.

6-25-16

Dr Edwards started me on Contrave to help stop my cravings and to continue or at least maintain weight loss.

Weight 319.4

Body Fat 51%

Muscle 30.9 pounds

Body water 38.7%

BMI 52.8

Nov. 12, 2016

My last total body weight composition at Dr. Edwards free clinic:

Weight 309.6 pounds

Body fat 51%

Body water 38.9%

Muscle 30.6 pounds

Fasting Glucose around this time was usually 142

I know the numbers above because Dr. Edwards set up a spreadsheet on google documents for me. He had me type my weight and fasting glucose everyday as he followed along on his computer.

I am grateful to Dr. Edwards treatment of me for one year.

Anonymous

PREFACE

Wake up call:

So much in the guidelines are wrong. Guidelines are usually considered the minimum to do.

Guidelines are still using LDLc levels instead of LDL particle count (LDLp).

NLA (National Lipid Association) has progressed to using non-HDL cholesterol goals which I proposed in my book, *The Tubby Theory from Topeka* back in 2009. Non-HDLc is all the cholesterol except the HDLc.

<u>Other mistakes in guidelines:</u>

1. Advising very expensive PCSK9 IV drug instead of using low dose inexpensive generic triple therapy to get to the very lowest LDLp. Triple therapy I advise is lowest dose of statin, ezetimibe and only 1,000 mg of Endur-acin (niacin). I found Endur-acin to be very effective with much less side effects than brand name niacin.
2. Taking in-expensive Niacin off the alternative drug list to statins. They made this decision due to data that turned out to not be significant after further analysis.
3. Not understanding the Sponge theory as a cause of the reduced obese re-gaining weight and advising diet and exercise as the way to continue to maintain weight loss despite this approach failed with the *Look Ahead trial.*
4. Believing the obese can "outrun their fork".
5. Thinking a calorie is a calorie.
6. Believing the reduced obese can maintain their weight with exercise.

I was reviewing the two best diet books of 2016: *Always Hungry* by David Ludwig and *The Change Your Biology Diet* by Louis J Aronne.

They are good diet books.

They reflect the change away from *low fat* diet books. These two books also reflect the general opinion that Atkins is too restrictive on carbohydrates and thus cannot be continued long term for more than 6-10 months.

Both books both put forth diets allowing more carbohydrates that have *low glycemic indexes. "This will slowly reprogram your fat cells,"* Dr. Ludwig claims.

My problem with this is I don't believe it affects the low leptin levels.

Dr. Aronne goes one step further with exercise. Claiming that 10 minutes twice a week of high intensity exercise will make the difference. HIs secret is to do the exercise till muscle failure.

My problem with this is it may lead to injuries especially in the elderly.

I suggest people do 3 sets of 25 repetitions low weights four days a week. This is done to preserve muscle mass with weight loss by also eating 2.4 gram protein/kg. lean body weight.

This is difficult, but probably easier than low repetitions with high weights. Start with one set the first week and then increase another two sets over two weeks. You will know the correct weight for you as the last three repetitions should burn your muscles.

After I passed the American Board of Obesity Medicine exam in December 2015, I was astonished that my Professors are selling the old diet and exercise routine. Dr Arrone has suggested multiple diet medications are the answer at Obesity meetings for some people.

We know from the failed *Look Ahead trial* that diet and exercise does not work over the long term. It was a negative trial and was stopped after 10 years due to futility.

Source:

Cardiovascular Effects of Intensive Lifestyle Intervention in Type 2 Diabetes

The Look AHEAD Research Group*

N Engl J Med 2013; 369:145-154 July 11, 2013DOI: 10.1056/NEJMoa1212914

In my preparation for the Obesity Boards, I went to several conferences. The Physicians with the most clinical experience taught that the guidelines are wrong. You cannot outrun your fork.

The guidelines tell the *reduced obese* that in order to maintain their weight loss they simply need to walk an hour a day and maintain 1200 to 1500 calorie diet a day. This is what people do who have maintained weight loss in the National Weight Control Registry (NCWR).

The American Board of Obesity Medicine (ABOM) lecturers pointed to the history of Ancel Keys *Great Starvation Experiment.* At the end of WWII, Dr. Keys put 32 conscientious objectors on a starvation diet and exercised them for 24 weeks.

They were on 1550 calories a day and walked an hour a day.

These men were so miserable many of them were eating garbage. When they were caught doing this infraction they were kicked out of the program in shame.

The guidelines expect our reduced obese patients to follow the same starvation level of calories and exercise for the rest of their lives just to maintain their weight loss. Ten thousand people in the NCWR(National Weight Control Registry) have said they are able to do it.

This starvation diet was also given to Prisoners of War during World War Two in Japan.

1.25 cup of white rice= 300 calories.

3 meals a day=1200 calories.

Not sure how many calories I should give the 400 cc of soup? 200 to 400 calories/d?

Source: WWII exhibit at Kansas State

Please go to my Blog site (The Tubby Traveler to Topeka)

meandgin.blogspot.com (my blog) to see a photo of the exhibit and the food given to the prisoners. In search type: Diet fed to WW Two prisoners of Japan

Blog address for WW Two prisoners

This information that you need to stay on a starvation diet just to maintain your weight loss has not truly been embraced by the nutrition obesity industry as they feel it is too dark. I faced a similar situation after I passed the Boards of the National Lipidology Association in 2007. Tim Russert had died and no lipidologist spoke out on National TV that he was not treated correctly according to guidelines. Thus I wrote *The Tubby Theory from Topeka*.

I coined the term *Tubby Factor* to replace the complicated term *non-HDL cholesterol (non-HDLc)*. Mr. Russert's non-HDLc was not at goal. I suspect his physician had no idea what that was. Certainly none of the cardiologists on TV ever mentioned it.

I also proposed a way to prevent the 100,000/yr sudden coronary deaths by getting a CAC (CT of heart) and/or CIMT (carotid intimal wall thickening ultrasoud) on every patient with one risk factor.

Interestingly, my ideas (which were taught to me by my Professors at the NLA) were validated by the latest AHA/ACA guidelines.

At the NLA Masters Program in New Orleans 2016, Dr. Jacobson looks at me during a class and says "we should call non-HDLc something different. Maybe non-LDL" I had given him a copy of my book when it first came out. I guess he forgot I already did this by suggesting we call non-HDL cholesterol the Tubby Factor, as most people with discordance (of LDLc vs. non-HDLc) have metabolic syndrome with large waists.

NLA recently replaced LDLc with non-HDLc (Tubby Factor) as the standard biomarker to use when treating patients. I predicted this in my book. I wrote I would have preferred they make LDLp or apoB the standard but I knew they could never get the consensus as most of the trial data used LDLc. Also non-HDLc can be calculated from the traditional lipid panel. Much cheaper than getting advanced lipid testing.

Once again after passing Boards in a new subject, Obesity, I see my Professors hedging their bets. I know, Dr. Aronne is holding back in his medication chapter because he taught me how to use diet medications. He said he uses multiple diet medications in some patients. No trials to support it works except with Contrave (naloxone/buspirone) and Qsymia (phentermine/topiramate). Many Doctors also are giving their diabetes type 2 patients metformin, invokana and lower dose liraglutide. No trials yet on patients who take 5 drugs, just experience among many diabetic patients who are also being treated for Obesity.

INTRODUCTION

People can't maintain their weight loss.

I maintained my eighty pound weight loss after giving up on extreme exercise and switching to Atkins ad libitum (eating till full) diet but more importantly in taking multiple diet medications.

Summary of my major weight loss with medications:

1. Invokana 300 mg 3-4-14 (262 lbs) to 6-24-15 (244 lbs)
2. Qsymia 6-24-15 (244 lbs) to 11-9-16 (213.4 lbs)
3. Belviq 10 mg BID 11-15-16 (212.4 lbs) to 3-1-17(212.4 lb)
4. Liraglutide to maximum dose for dieting 3.0 mg on 3-1-17 (212.4 lbs. on HAWAII SCALE) to (200.8 lbs on Topeka scale).

It was also very important to stop Insulin and Actos for my weight loss. These two drugs cause weight gain.

The multiple diet medicines have helped me maintain my weight loss from 280 lbs to 200 lbs from Feb 2006 till *12 years later.*

I think Atkins was essential as I ate ad libitum(essentially this means eat till you are full) and *was never hungry.* This is the type of diet I could eat for the rest of my life. I didn't really lose weight on Atkins, I mostly stopped gaining weight even though I decreased my exercise from 2 hours a day to walking 20-40 minutes a day. I documented my weight maintenance of 246 lbs during 2011 as I went on cruises and traveling around the world in my book, *The Tubby Traveler from Topeka.*

I lost significant weight when I added Invokana(canagliflozin). Invokana is indicated for diabetes. I used it to replace Insulin in my type 2 Diabetes Mellitus. Invokana causes approximately 200 calories of glucose to be lost in the urine each day. My last Hgb. A1c was 6.7 on 6-6-17.

Not everyone will lose weight with Invokana. I was also taking Victoza 1.8 mg. at the time.

I later started Qsymia and after 16 months I replaced it with Belviq.

The diet medicines circumvented the Sponge syndrome (caused by very high number of fat cells retained from my peak weight 280 lbs).

I maintained a 30 pound weight loss from Jan. 2011 with Atkins ad libitum and 20-40 minutes walking.

From June 24, 2015 I lost another 44 lbs by adding Qsymia and later switching to Belviq and increasing my Liraglutide dose to 3.0 mg a day.

This is the message my book is going to convey.

It's all about finding a diet you can stay on for life and the medication you will need as weight regain occurs due to Sponge Syndrome.

ABBREVIATIONS

OBESITY SCIENCE TERMS

MiRNA: Micro RNA (small non-coding RNA)

NPY/AgRP neurons: activated by Ghrelin.
(Ghrelin stimulate NPY release and AgRP release increase orexigenic pathway.)

MSH: melanocyte stimulating hormone
VMH: ventromedial hypothalamus
POMC: proopiomelanocortin

LCHF: low carbohydrate high fat

MEDICAL IMAGING

CIMT: Carotid Intimal Wall Thickening (it is an ultrasound test)

CAC: Coronary artery calcium (measured on a CT scan of heart)

BLOOD TESTS

LDL: low density lipoprotein

LDLc: specifically LDL cholesterol (usually is calculated)

LDLp: specifically LDL particle

HDL: high density lipoprotein

non-HDLc: all the cholesterol without the HDLc

ASSOCIATIONS:

NLA: National Lipid Association
NLAF: Fellow of National Lipid Association7

DIABETES

IR: insulin resistance

CHOLESTEROL LOWERING DRUG

PCSk-9:Proprotein convertase subtilisin/kexin (is an enzyme encoded by the *PCSK9* gene
PCSK-9 inhibitor: a new type of drug (such as alirocumab)that binds the protein, *paradoxically,* you lower cholesterol.
PCSK-9 destroys the liver *PCSK9 receptor.*
Normally the PCSK-9 receptor clears cholesterol to be destroyed and recycled hence the word paradoxical.

CHRONOLOGY

My Chronic Obesity Weight Record

9-1960	115 lbs	Second grade Age 9
8-31-1964	150 lbs	5 ft 5" Age 12
	(BMI 25 95%tile on growth chart)	
9-19-1965	175 lbs	5 ft 8.5" Age 13
	(BMI 26 95th %tile on growth chart)	
10-30-1967	185 lbs	5'9" Age 15
	(started Weight Watchers Diet)	
4-68	160 lbs	5'10"
	(16 yrs 70th %tile on growth chart)	
6-30-69	166 lbs	waist 33.5"
6-17-1970	173 lbs	5'11" 19yrs
	BMI 24	waist 35"

7-2-1970	164 lbs.	34" waist
	Ran mile in 5 min 20 seconds	
12-5-1972	1-171973	200 lbs
		180 lbs
1-10-1974	194 lbs	38.25" waist

1988

I went from 245 pounds to 208 pounds.

My first big weight loss while working at my first medical practice in Clermont, Fl.

I attended Overeaters Anonymous Meetings.

I went to Nautilus weights 3 times a week and jogged daily while on 1,000 calories. I stayed at this weight for a few months but the deprivation was too much and I quickly went up to 220 pounds.

10-1995	272 lbs	49" waist
	I could bench press 340 pounds free weight.	
	(I went on Fastin and Pondimin.)	
1996	*220 lbs,*	*Waist 42" Age 45*
1998	240 lbs,	Age 47

Feb 2006
280 lbs

Nov 2006
200 lbs

Dec 2010
250 lbs

March 1, 2014
265 lbs
I started Invokana and stopped Insulin.
My glucose immediately improved going down below 150.
I went down to 239.5 lbs without changing diet or exercise

6-25-15
244.8 lbs,
Waist 43"
(Weigh in at Stormont Vail Obesity Clinic)

(Started Qsymia lost 21 lbs)

11-15-16
212.4
Switched to Belviq 10 mg BID)
I had to stop Qsymia due to fast heart rate.
I did not lose more weight with Belviq but I achieved my goal to maintain my weight loss.)

3-1-17
212.4 lb
I changed my Victoza (liraglutide) dose 1.8 mg (DM dose) to Saxenda (liraglutide) dose 3.0 (diet dose) on first day of Hawaii vacation as I was told I had to lose (incorrectly) another 5% to be allowed to stay on the diet drugs.

5-31-17
203 LBS
I went back to the diabetic dose of Victoza 1.8 mg. (diabetic dose for liraglutide)

7-27-17
199 lbs.

12-10-17
214.4 lbs
Increased Victoza from 1.8 to Saxenda dose 3.0 (diet dose for liraglutide)

1-5-2018
203.2 lbs
Decreased Victoza to 1.8 mg (diabetic dose)

PART ONE

CHRONIC OBESITY

MY CHRONIC OBESITY (PHOTOS)

I always thought I was a chubby child. I tried to pull up some photos to document it.

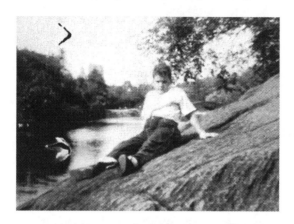

July-1958
Age 7 yrs 7 mos
Summer in Central Park, NYC I was called "husky" size at this age.

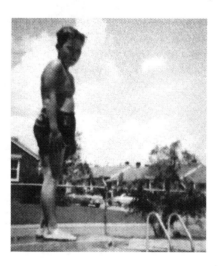

August 1960.
9 years 8 months. I was a big kid for my age.
I thought I was overweight. I ate a tremendous amount and was very active.
Finished second grade.

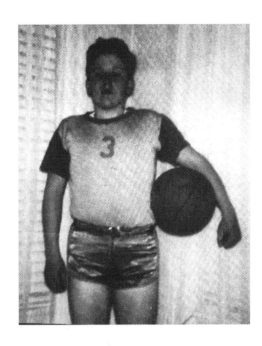

10-1963
12 years 10 months.
Sixth grade at Public School 89 in Brooklyn, NY)

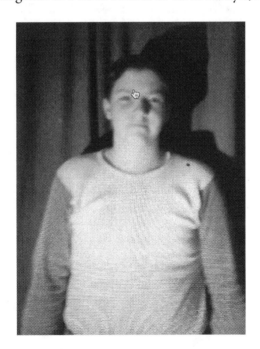

4-1965
Age 14 years 4 months
Seventh grade at Andreas Hudde High School on school basketball team
Went on Weight Watchers Diet in High School.

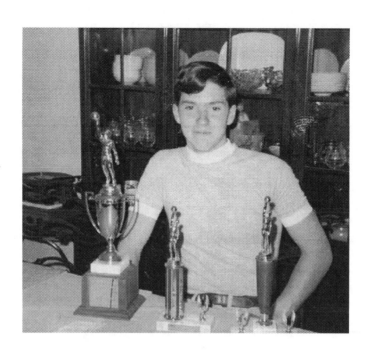

April 1968
Age 17 yrs 4 mos
I am at 5'10 and 160 lbs
Junior at Stuyvesant High School in Manhattan, NYC
To get to this weight I had been on Weight Watchers.

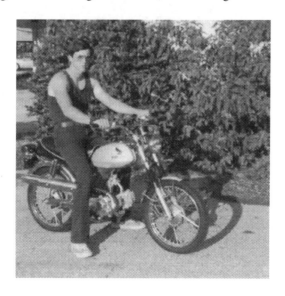

July 1970
Age 19 yrs 7 mos
After my first year at Brooklyn College

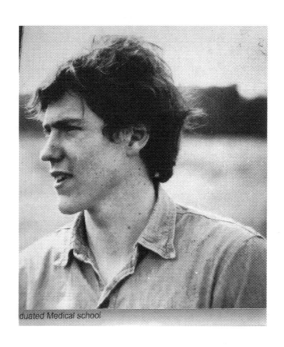

August 1972
Age 21 years 8 mos
Taken in Richmond Park, England

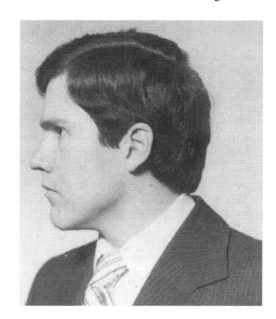

June 1977
Age 26 yrs 6 mos
Graduated Medical school

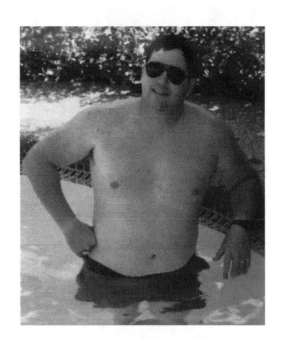

July 1988
Age 37
245 lbs

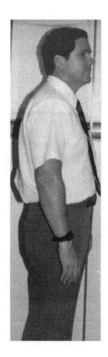

Sept. 1989
208 lbs
Age 38

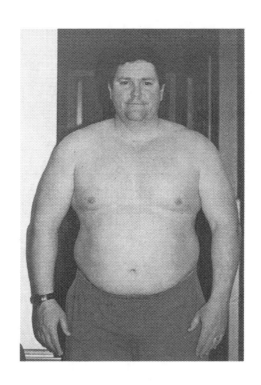

10-95
Age 44
272 lbs
Waist 49"

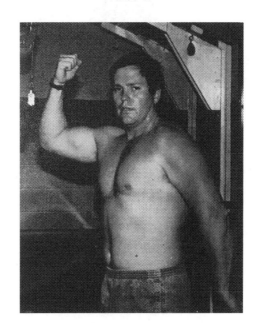

Nov. 1996
Age 45
220 lbs
Waist 42"

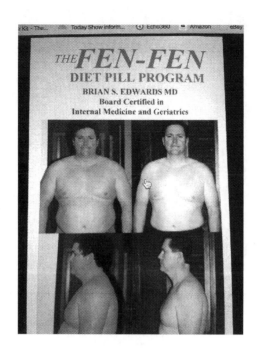

Dec 1996

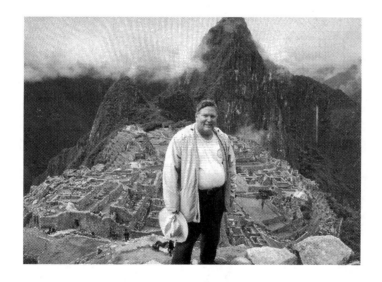

Dec 2005
280 lbs
Age 54
March 2006 I started *The 3 Hour Diet* by Jorge Cruise

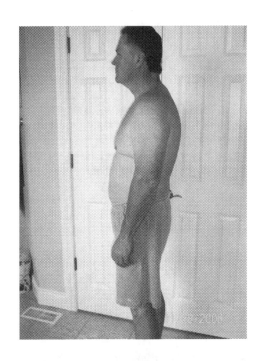

11-28-2006
200 lbs
Age 55

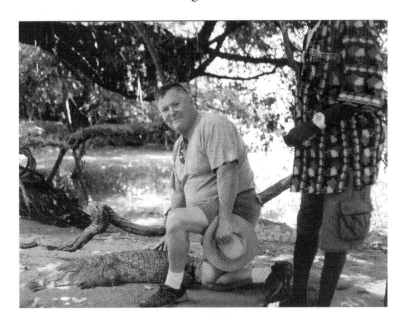

11-27-2010
Age 58
250 lbs

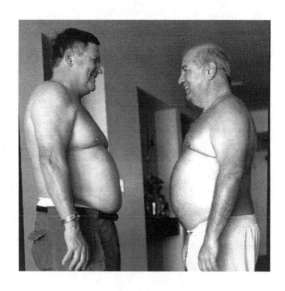

2-24-11
Age 59
After being on Atkins diet for one month.
No change in weight over that month.

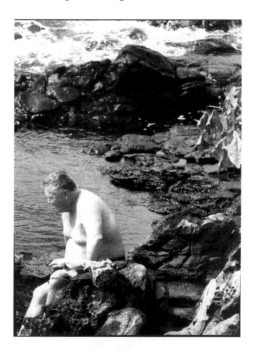

Jan 2014
Age 63
260 lbs
I started Invokana and stopped Insulin in March 2014
My glucose immediately improved going down below 150.

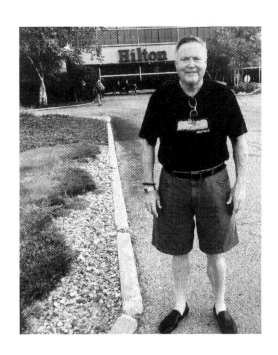

August 2014
Age 63
239.5 lbs without changing diet or exercise

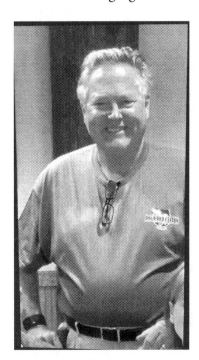

6-16-15
244.8 lbs,
Waist 43"
Weigh in at Stormont Vail Obesity Clinic
Started Qsymia 6-24-15

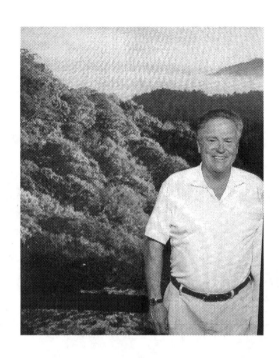

11-7-2016
213.6 lbs
Switched to Belviq on 11-15-16

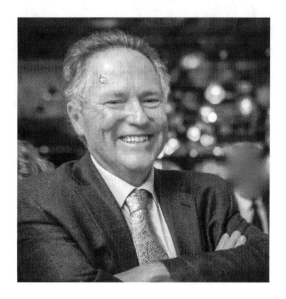

5-12-17
Age 65
203.6 lbs
Wedding in Philadelphia

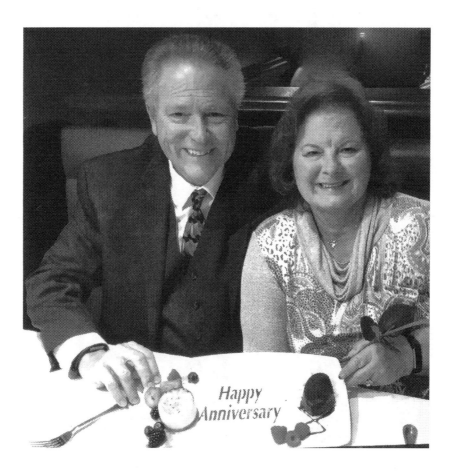

12-13-17
208.4
Having a great meal the Capital Grill at the Plaza, Kansas City

1

HOW TO MAINTAIN WEIGHT LOSS.

To maintain your weight loss <u>you must stay on your reduced calorie diet for life,</u> especially when you hit your plateau after 6-9 months.

That could be the end of this book. It is dark news.

In the National Weight Control Registry (NWCR) there are 10,000 people who have maintained their weight loss over more than five years. They stay on low calorie diets ranging from 1200 to 1500 calories and walk an hour a day.

That is what works.

So do it, the guidelines say. It's all about willpower to maintain the lifestyle?

I don't understand why the guidelines discount the chemical pathways between gut, fat and brain that cause weight regain because the body thinks it is starving. Leptin, Insulin, and Ghrelin are the big three.

The good news is there are diet medications to help control the hunger when you hit your plateau and the Sponge syndrome kicks in. However, the media and most Doctors have not embraced this good news yet.

These are good books for losing weight.

1. *The New Atkins for a New You* by Westman, Phinney and Votek 2010
2. *Always Hungry?* by David Ludwig MD, PhD
3. *Change Your Biology Diet* by Louis J. Aronne MD
4. *South Beach Diet* by Arthur Agatston MD
5. *The Diet Fix. Why diets fail and how to make yours work* by Yoni Freedhoff.
6. *New Hippocratic Diet guide* by Dr Irving A. Cohen

The problem is reading them and following them.

None of them have data that their diet keeps the weight off.

My book documents my 80 pound weight loss maintained over 11 years. Case study number of one.

I ate Atkins ad libitum(I ate till I was full) and was not hungry while walking 20 to 40 minutes/day. I drank alcohol. The diet medications were the key to success.

In this book I show my personal history at maintaining weight loss:

March 2006 I was 280 pounds

June 2017. I was 200 lbs

First rule: Keep it simple.

Keeping diaries for the rest of your life is not simple.

Counting calories is not simple.

I suspect the reduced obese that read this book have used diaries and calorie counting with short term effectiveness.

The books mentioned above, in large part, are all different versions of the low carbohydrate high fat diet.

They usually include "phases".

These are too complicated for most patients.

I truly doubt they make a difference in the long run for 90% of the reduced obese who are trying to maintain their weight loss.

The phases are an attempt by the authors to get back to a less restrictive diet for life. If that means more calories, the reduced obese will gain weight.

All the books listed above include recipes.

I have never made a meal from any of these books' recipes.

For those people who use these books as guides and have succeeded, I congratulate them and admire them. Actually half of the people in NWCR have maintained their weight loss completely on their own. The people with this amazing will power are the people scientists want in their trials. It appears all weight loss diets or surgery have "waterfall"results. This means there a wide range of weight loss results in both the tested group and the control group.

I will talk about the *LOOK AHEAD* trial later. The best and biggest scientific effort to prove diet and exercise will work over the long run to lower cardiovascular events. It failed.

Why? Probably because the people in the control group were just as mentally and psychologically capable of doing it on their own in the long run. The waterfall results were very similar in both groups. After 4 years there was only a 3.6% difference in weight loss between the control and the treatment group.

(Reference for Waterfall results see my Blog *The Tubby Traveler from Topeka* and search Waterfall results. *http://meandgin.blogspot.com/search?q=waterfall+results*)

In the practice of Clinical Obesity, we don't get to choose our patients.

Our patients want a magical pill that makes them lose weight that doesn't cost much and no side effects.

Unfortunately the patients still don't want to continue diet medications after they lose their weight because the patients consider it a crutch or it costs too much money.

Gastric Bypass surgery is now seen as that magic procedure for many. At one of my Obesity conferences, a slide showed that 30% of bariatric surgery patients gain their weight back after 10 years. A recent article showed 20% of bariatric patients are on pain medications after several years.

THE CHRONIC DISEASE OF OBESITY

I was 280 pounds in March 2006 and lost 80 pounds in time for my wedding in June 2007. I did it the old fashion way by counting calories and exercising one to two hours a day. *(The Three Hour Diet* by Jorge Cruise)

I was exhausted by the discipline and always hungry despite 5 meals a day. I decided to eat more fruit and increase my exercise to 2 hours 30 minutes a day. I gained 1.5 pounds a month till I had a re-gain of 50 pounds by 2011. I realize now my big mistake was to eat "healthy fruit" or low glycemic fruit. Instead of fruit for my mid-morning and mid-afternoon snacks, I should have had a minimum of 10 grams of protein for each snack.

I suggest a protein drink such as

1. *Protein Premier* 30 grams of protein at 160 calories or (3g fat)
2. *Atkins shake* 15 grams of protein with 160 calories. (9g fat)
3. depending on the amount of exercise you do, but especially for intense weightlifters try:
4. *EAS MYO* 42g protein, 300 calories, 7g fat.
   People trying to get into a nutritional ketosis state may want more fat.
5. Premier Protein *Clear Protein Drink. 20 g protein 90 calories 0 sugar I add this to Powerade Zero Fruit Punch to cut the sweetness.*

Now that I am back down to 200 lbs I plan to follow a protein diet of 150-180 grams a day with a weight lifting program of 25 repetitions 3 sets at least 4 times a week. Elderly men develop a condition called *sarcopenia* which is loss of muscle mass, mostly in the legs. I try to lift weights everyday, alternating upper body on even days and lower body on odd days. My appetite does increase with this. I feel full but the desire for certain foods continues. I have found my one cup of caffeinated coffee in the afternoon helps. Certainly the diet medications prevent my hunger but not always the craving that may come with boredom of a restrictive diet.

If you can keep carbs down to six days a week and not binge on them, the Atkins might still work for you.

I know if I bring ice cream into the house or a whole pizza, I can't limit my portions.

If I don't eat high protein (30 grams or more) breakfast, lunch and dinner I get very hungry between meals. When I do get hungry between meals I eat a protein snack that has at least 10 grams of protein. Atkins French Vanilla shake is 160 cal, 2g CHO (carbs), and 15 grams protein. I also eat Almonds or Pistachios.

Even with the high protein diet, the more I exercise I do the more hungry I get.

I found diet medication clearly allowed me to eat less on the same Atkins diet and exercise yet still lose weight. Diet medication has also allowed me to not regain on same diet and exercise without increased hunger.

At the Obesity Teaching Courses from TOS The Obesity Society) in Orlando, Fl. in 2011, I learned about:

1. Leptin,
2. the Reduced obese state, and
3. the billions of fat cells that remain despite my 80 pound weight loss

I was writing my book, *The Tubby Traveler from Topeka* and subsequently elucidated the *Sponge Syndrome theory.*

Weight loss from diet,exercise or bariatric surgery cause billions of fat cells to shrink *but not to disappear* and continue to produce less leptin.

Patients gain fat even at low level of calories and high levels of exercise as the body thinks it is starving. Diet, exercise or Bariatric surgery do not reduce the *number* of fat cells, they only *shrink* them with weight loss.

The Biggest Loser experiment (see Gina Kolata's NYT article on 5-1-16
: *After 'The Biggest Loser,' Their Bodies Fought to Regain)* has recently validated my theory. It's not the amount of lean muscle loss that causes the weight regain, it is the amount of fat lost with the resultant low level of Leptin in all the remaining fat cells. The best way to prevent weight regain in the *Reduced Obese* is to address this low Leptin level with multiple diet medications.

Before we get to the diet medications, in order to *maintain weight loss* the patient has to:

1. find a *restrictive diet* he/she can maintain for the rest of their life. It must be low (1,000-2,000/d) in calories for the rest of their lives.
2. Weigh every day (Very Important)
3. Walk 20 minutes a day for health not weight loss
4. Expect weight loss for only 6-9 months
5. At plateau, don't expect to break through with lower calories or more exercise or even diet medications.

After hitting the plateau with the diet that has worked for you in the past, I would advise those people who are not on a Atkins type diet which is LCHF (low carbohydrate high fat diet) to switch to LCHF diet.

Reasons for switch at plateau:

1. No calorie counting
2. Just don't eat carbohydrates
3. LCHF (Atkins) is ad libitum(you eat till you are full)

You avoid hunger because of high protein and nutritional ketosis, thus you are satisfied with 500 less calories. (the challenge is to stop eating when you are full)

4. LCHF (Atkins) tastes good because of high fat.

At the plateau, the *goal* is simply to feel satisfied with the restrictive diet and not gain weight.

If there is significant weight regain, it is time for diet medications or to add more diet medications.

LCHF diet and the diet medications are for the rest of your life.

THE CHRONIC DISEASE OF OBESITY

If you are not prepared to take diet medications for the rest of your life, you probably should not bother to start.

This is the treatment of the Chronic Disease of Obesity.

If you do better with another diet and can stay on it for life, then by all means use what works especially if you are not diabetic type 2, pre-diabetic or don't have the metabolic syndrome

Multiple diet medications: Contrave, Qsymia are combination medication that are on label. However it is very easy to go off label with diet medications as the physician individualizes treatment.

Off label means using medications to treat disorders not listed under FDA indications listed in PDR (physicians desk reference)

FDA anti-obesity medication indications:

1. BMI (Body mass index) greater than or equal to 30kg/m^2
2. BMI greater than or equal to 27 kg/m^2 with presence of
    Diabetes mellitus
    Hypertension
    Dyslipidemia

In Kansas, the Stormont Obesity Clinic told me I had to lose 5% of my weight in order to be allowed to take the diet medication for the rest of my life.

For the reduced obese at plateau this may not be feasible.

They need the diet medications not to lose more weight but to maintain their weight.

If you are worried you cannot lose another five percent of weight after already hitting the plateau, start a very high protein diet with weight lifting. Gain 5-10 lbs of muscle and it may be possible to lose another 5% on the new diet pill. Hopefully you can keep the muscle gain by continuing high protein 2.4 g/kg and high reps with low weight resistance training 4 days a week.

I believe the Federal guidelines simply want clinical improvement shown rather than precisely 5% weight loss. If your osteoarthritis pain is less, that is a clinical improvement.

If a patient has tolerated a diet medicine for 12 weeks and had some intermittent benefit as I did with Liraglutide(Victoza), don't give up on it. Adding Qsymia to the Victoza made a tremendous difference to my program.

I was on six diet medications but I switched from Qsymia to Belviq and am now on 5 diet medications.

1. Metformin
2. Invokana
3. Victoza
4. Qsymia (phentermine/topiramate)
5.   caffeine (coffee)
6.   Belviq (Locaserin)

I am also on ad libitum Atkins diet and usually have a serum nutritional ketosis with ketone level greater than 0.5.

I call my diet the *Bon Vivant diet* because I go on cruises and drink alcohol daily.

I only walk 1-2 miles a day. (recently added weight lifting)

Easy to be "off label" on diet medications:

I went to a Saxenda presentation recently and to my amazement I learned I am supposed to increase the dose every week without fail till the maximum dose.

If the patient cannot tolerate the maximum dose they have to give up on the drug.

They can't go back to the lower dose without side effects that may have had an effective weight loss of 5%? No?

However if the patient tolerates the high dose and loses weight, the patient can cut Saxenda down to a lower dose if they wish.

The reader will learn while reading this book that Victoza (which I take) and Saxenda (comes in higher doses) are exactly the same drug (Liraglutide).

Saxenda has a 40% side effect report. Despite this high rate of side effects most people are able to tough through the nausea and stay on the drug.

I had abdominal pain on Victoza. I backed off for a while and returned to it more slowly. A physician has to be allowed to treat patients on an individual basis.

Your physician may ask you to sign a document realizing you are taking a drug off label (using a drug for something not indicated in Physicians Desk Reference (PDR) Using drugs off label is very common but releases from patients usually are not asked for by the Doctor.

2

FOUR SIMPLE IDEAS

THE TOPEKA TUBBY DIET IN 4 STEPS

1.   You can't outrun your fork

Exercise to maintain weight loss is not a good long term strategy because it is usually not sustainable long term.

Injury, life events, and weather often interfere with continuing a strenuous exercise program. Weight regain will occur as the diet is already at a moderate calorie level in order to sustain the exercise or to prevent more hunger that comes with more exercise.

Once your exercise decreases you must go to lower calories.

In the Sponge syndrome this is very insidious over a period of years. Minor lapses will cause surprising weight gain.

A better strategy is to exercise less on a daily basis in a way that comes naturally no matter what the circumstances of life. A twenty minute walk a day is sustainable once incorporated into the day. Then if weight regain starts to creep in, there is more exercise that can be turned to on an intermittent basis to lose those 3-5 extra pounds as well as use meal replacement to make certain overeating is not an issue.

The Reduced obese have a 42% reduction in their exercise metabolism.

This means a mile walk does not burn 100 calories, it only burns 58 calories. This adds a tremendous burden of time onto what is already a difficult and challenging program just to maintain the reduc*ed weight.*

2.   Best Bang for Buck for health is 20 minute walk

No question that exercise is the fountain of youth if not overdone. It is a poor strategy for weight loss however. Large weight loss usually occurs with muscle loss. Some strategies suggest that high protein weight loss diet with resistance training can prevent the muscle loss.

(see *A Diet and Exercise Plan to Lose Weight and Gain Muscle -* Gretchen Reynolds https:// well.blogs.nytimes.com/.../a-diet-and-exercise-plan-to-lose-weight-and-gain-m...

Feb 3, 2016

There was a belief that muscle turned into fat in muscle men. I think those men engaged in high level exercise with high calorie intake. At some point the intense exercise stopped but the intense food intake did not. Thus these muscle men became overweight.

Muscles burn a small percentage of the total metabolism.

Only athletes at very high levels of intense performance make a big difference. Marathon runners for example. High intensity exercise for one hour can burn 600 calories. The problem is exercise metabolism is reduced by 38% after you lose 10% of your weight.

Resistance training is a good idea as the muscles protect your joints from injury.

Exercise for health not weight loss.

Don't overdo it (exercise) as this has sabotaged many diet programs.

3.   **Weight loss usually occurs over first 6-9 months then plateau and regain**

(Reference for this is at my blog: http://meandgin.blogspot.com/search?q=plateau
Or go to my blog *The Tubby Traveler from Topeka* and search *plateau*.)

This is the problem.

Why don't the other diet books emphasize this?

They instead talk about breaking through the plateau.

If with monumental effort a person does break through the plateau it does not persist, weight regain will occur due to low Leptin level due to shrunken fat cells that NEVER DISAPPEAR. *The Sponge Syndrome*. I have broken through three plateaus at 240 lbs, 220 lbs and 210 lbs. I did it while following the same diet and exercise. I did by eating less to be full on multiple diet medications.

To obtain the initial weight loss, *virtually any low calorie diet is acceptable.*

Then at the plateau in 6-9 months I would suggest switching to a ad libitum (eat till you are full) diet so that the diet does not feel quite so restrictive for the rest of the patient's life and to prevent hunger.

I myself switched to Atkins and stopped the regain despite decreasing my exercise from 2.5 hours a day to 20 minutes a day and I happily ate ad libitum on cruises. However, I did not lose weight. I never documented myself to be in nutritional ketosis by urine check. I suspect it is because I did eat large amounts of food. Later I started checking my blood ketones with a finger stick. I found I was in nutritional ketosis and yet not losing weight. Low Leptin still trumps ketones, exercise and high protein diet to cause hunger and physiologic changes to prevent starvation. I believe the excess number of fat cells cause more MiRNA's to be secreted by these shunken fats with a low leptin level.

Hence the next unavoidable necessary step.

4.   **Diet medications (multiple if needed)**

The best way to treat low Leptin levels is multiple diet medications that fool multiple brain pathways that enables the brain to gain weight despite exercise and low calorie levels. When the Leptin level is low the brain believes the body is starving even though the patient is not at his optimum BMI(weight).

This is why two diet pills are a combination of two diet medicines:

Qsymia (phentermine/topiramate)

Contrave (naltrexone/bupropion)

The brain usually outsmarts phentermine after 9 months of use.

Belviq is only one drug: Locaserin (it is similar to the old fenfluramine that caused heart valve problems and caused the Phentermine/Fenfluramine combination to be taken off the market.)

One trial showed 50% of dieters don't respond to Belviq. If there is no weight loss I would suggest adding Phentermine at it's lowest dose. This is off label but is similar to the old Phen-Fen diet pill that was very effective.

Rather than put a patient on high dose Saxenda which is around $1,000 a month as most insurance doesn't cover it, I put the patient on Victoza if they have diabetes type ll and then it is covered by insurance. Metformin is also covered by insurance and may also help weight loss. Replacing insulin with Invokana worked very well with me.

3

FOUR NEW DIET MEDICATIONS

Presently there are four new drugs for long term treatment of chronic obesity.

If there is an epidemic of obesity why is it not being treated with medications?

As a Diplomat of the American Board of Obesity Medicine and a Fellow and Diplomat in the National Lipid Association I think physicians should consider putting their obese patients on one of the following diet medicines for the chronic disease of obesity on a long term basis:

1. Lorcaserin (BELVIQ)
2. Phentermine/Topiramate (QSYMIA)
3. Liraglutide (SAXENDA)
4. Naltrexone/Bupropion (CONTRAVE)

My personal experience is with Victoza, Invokana and Qsymia and Belviq. These medications are available only with a physician's prescription. Belviq and Qsymia are controlled substances and require a physician's DEA number.

Let me give some ideas as to how to choose which drug, *which must be done in concert with your physician.*

Diet meds usually indicated if BMI >26 + comorbidity or > 30.

First step.

If fasting glucose >99 go on Metformin. This blood sugar levels means the patient has pre-diabetes.

Second step.

If diabetic already and is on maximum dose Metformin, add Victoza as this low dose(1.8 mg.) Liraglutide will be paid for by insurance.

Third step.

If on Insulin try switching over to Invokana. Careful monitoring of glucose during transition and suggest switching to Atkins or any LCHF (low carbohydrate high fat diet).

Now for the Diet medicines themselves.

First choice?

LOCASERIN (Belviq)
Scheduled drug. (Needs your physician's DEA number)
May be safest drug.
Young women are less of a concern for side effects than with Qsymia.
Caution with depressed patients.
There is a concern for *serotonin syndrome* but to my knowledge this drug does not increase serotonin levels.
Downside: Only 50% have good response.
Solution: After two or three months add Phentermine one half tab 37.5 mg a day if no cardiac or anxiety contraindications. This is generic drug now. This addition is off label for long term despite the combination in Qsymia having the indication for long term.

Second choice?

PHENTERMINE/TOPIRAMATE (QSYMIA)
Scheduled drug. (Needs your physician's DEA number)
Main concern: REMS caution for pregnancy testing.
Good point: Can give to depressed patients.
Side-effects: high dose can cause problems with cognition and dysgeusia (bad taste) especially with diet soda.
Potentiates alcohol.
Metabolic acidosis, decrease potassium, increase creatinine.
Consider getting blood chemistry level after first month of treatment.

Third Choice?

NALTREXONE/BUPROPION (CONTRAVE)
Best news: Non-scheduled drug
Bad news: *Label legacy*
These 2 drugs have been around for so long that many side effects have shown up in the PDR(physician desk reference) over the years.
BLACK BOX WARNING: Depression and Neuro-psych disorders
Do not give to people on narcotic pain medicine.
Careful in people prone to seizures.

Thus in young folks who might binge on alcohol this might not be the first choice.

Not for bulimia or anorexia nervosa

Don't take with Levadopa or Amantadine

UPDATE: Still some concerns about increase HTN (hypertension or high blood pressure)? Constipation tends to occur with weight loss but seems more so with Contrave.

Fourth Choice?

LIRAGLUTIDE (Saxenda)

Expensive and is an injection.

If diabetic, can get lower dose paid for as Victoza.

BLACK BOX WARNING: Thyroid C cell tumors

Side effects: vomiting, pancreatitis, abdominal pain.

Despite 40% of people complain of side effects but they usually tough usually tough it out and stay on it.

Good news: Non-scheduled drug(only need Doctor's prescription, don't need his DEA number)

Frank Greenway recent review of Obesity Medicine :

"Following gastric bypass surgery, levels of ghrelin are extremely low, while GLP-1 and PYY are elevated, which should attenuate appetite."

International Journal of Obesity (2015) 39, 1188–1196; doi:10.1038/ijo.2015.59; published online 26 May 2015

Choosing which weight loss surgery is best for a patient is not based on random controlled double blind trials. Lap band was the most popular but doesn't work as well in the long term because it is not a bypass surgery. It only restricts the amount of food in the stomach.

The surgeons are allowed the freedom to discover the best course for the obese patients, while medical physicians face possible state retribution while finding the best diet medicine combination for their patients.

ABOM (American Board Obesity Medicine) specialists need to be allowed to use the best off-label treatment with multiple drugs to block the multiple pathways of starvation prevention that cause weight regain.

Use of multiple drugs that are off label is already being done to treat Diabetes Mellitus type 2, high blood pressure and infectious disease.

When Leptin is low it does not inhibit Ghrelin, thus Ghrelin is activated and increases hunger.

Leptin and Insulin share the same central feeding inhibitory and thermogenic pathways.

Peripherally, Insulin is <u>anabolic</u>

1. stores fat in adipose
2. stores glycogen in muscle and liver

Centrally, insulin is <u>catabolic</u> (as is Leptin)

1. breaks down molecules to release energy

In insulin resistance is seen in the following categories:

1. prediabetes (fasting glucose 100 or greater)
2. metabolic syndrome (waist greater than 40" causing high visceral fat)
3. diabetes mellitus type 2.

IR (insulin resistance) impairs capacity of the insulin receptor to signal the fat cell to halt triglyceride breakdown by Lipase and increases glucose uptake by glucose transport proteins. This increases release of fatty acids into central circulation and decreased uptake of glucose by fat cells.

4

NO FALSE HOPE HERE

Gina Kolata introduced me to the idea of false hope in her book *Rethinking thin*. I quote many of her chapters in my book, *The Tubby Traveler from Topeka in 2011.*

The idea that diet and exercise alone will maintain weight loss is still being advised in the guidelines. This is a false hope that is achieved by very few in the National Weight Control Registry. The people in NWCR are maintaining a 1200 to 1500 calorie diet and one hour exercise a day. Amazing people.

This is a sub-starvation diet just to maintain weight loss.

The reason it's not a starvation diet is that the low leptin levels prevent starvation with the Sponge syndrome.

The reduced obese must find a (restrictive) diet they can stay on for the rest of their lives.

A bad diet (high density carbohydrate foods in large quantities) will sabotage any diet even on diet medications, strenuous exercise or post bariatric surgery. We are indefensible against unlimited M&M's candy or excess alcohol (ETOH)

The key to a sustainable diet is to not be hungry.

More exercise makes you more hungry.

This is why more exercise is not the answer to maintaining weight loss, unless you maintain the same 1200 to 1500 calories a day as the people in NWCR do. When the volunteers in the Great Starvation diet did this for 24 weeks they suffered terribly. Dr Aronne believes his intense exercise will not have this effect, as it is only 10 minutes 2 times a week? We will see how it works out for his patients. However, to exercise to muscle failure is much too intense for most patients and will cause injury in my opinion.

Atkins (ad libitum) and Very Low calorie diets (800-1,000 calories) state that the subsequent *nutritional ketosis* these diets cause results in less appetite. As with many attempts(high protein and nutritional ketosis) to decrease hunger, eventually a diet medication should be added after nine to twelve months, when body will compensate with more hunger as the brain thinks it is starving because of the low leptin level.

Ludwig in *Always Hungry* believes that low glycemic carbohydrates will not stimulate insulin release which results in less hunger.

Bariatric surgery (excluding lap band) does not really work on restricting food amount. It works on hormonal changes in the gut that tells your brain you are full.

Sadly, these are all short term solutions when looking at 10 year data.

30% of people gain their weight back 10 years after bariatric surgery.

5

THE SCIENCE OF OBESITY

Insulin is probably one of the main reasons people gain their weight back from the plateau of weight loss.

Let me go through the physiology.

Insulin peripherally is anabolic. It promotes constructive metabolism. Insulin will store fat in adipose and glycogen in muscle and liver.

Insulin centrally is catabolic. (like Leptin) Insulin breaks down molecules to release energy.

Low Leptin increases food intake and suppresses energy expenditure. (Youdim p6).

"Leptin is an important signal for starvation."

High Leptin reduces food intake by inhibiting NPY/AgRP neurons and stimulating the alpha-MSH neurons. (Except in the Obese who become Leptin resistant. Only lean individuals appear to be regulating body weight.)

Centrally, Leptin and Insulin share same *feeding inhibitory and thermogenic* pathways.

However, in *Obese*, Insulin triggers steroidogenic factor 1 (SF-1) expressing neurons of the VMH, resulting in inhibition of POMC neurons, which promotes food intake and perpetuates obesity.

Let me repeat.

In lean individuals who have never been obese, leptin and insulin prevent them from becoming obese.

Centrally high levels of leptin and insulin reduce food intake and suppress energy expenditure through same pathway. Centrally both insulin and leptin are catabolic.

A lean individual eats a large meal. High insulin from pancreas peripherally stores fat and adipose and centrally increases thermogenesis to burn excess calories to maintain weight.

A "genetically obese prone" individual with early insulin resistance and early leptin resistance does all this less effectively.

Storing more fat, burning less energy and allowing more food intake on the slippery slope of always more appetite and more fat with more leptin and insulin resistance.

With tremendous will power an obese person follows the 3500 calorie rule to lose one pound of weight and is able to lose weight for 6-9 months until the plateau is reached.

At this point the thermodynamic laws of physics fail and the biological laws of survival take over.

Your body thinks you are starving. The plethora of retained fat cells in the reduced obese tell the brain this early warning.

The numerous fat cells did not disappear, they are shrunken. The subsequent low leptin level in the face of so many fat cells signals the body that starvation is occurring and MiRNA's are released.

This is the Sponge Syndrome.

So many fat cells remain in the reduced obese, so little leptin. Insulin probably high, but there is resistance to it's glucose lowering effect. MiRNA's are sent from the fat cells to all the body via blood stream.

Priority number one for the body is no longer to heat the body in order to restore the prior size of the fat cells.

Thermogenesis is reduced in the plateau as the determined dieter goes to 800 calories a day or increases to three hours of walking a day.

The physics of 3500 calories to lose one pound of weight fails.

This is where the dieter learns that most of calories burned during 24 hours are from the resting metabolism. Up to 70% of calories may be burned by the brain, liver, kidneys, heart, lungs, endocrine organs? Muscles themselves become food at this point, not the tool for a weight lifter to lose weight.

Thermogenesis is reduced by Leptin and Insulin and I suspect MiRNA

The dieter can do nothing about this.

Maybe the new diet pills and gastric bypass help?

Introducing Ghrelin.

The only hormone that stimulates appetite?

Leptin inhibits Ghrelin but not in obese.

Insulin inhibits Ghrelin centrally but not in obese.

The reduced obese with the billions of excess shrunken fat cells and subsequent low leptin level have Ghrelin levels making us thinking of nothing but our next meal.

The sub-starvation state. This miserable psychological condition is what most diet planners are telling us we must stay in to maintain our weight loss and they are wrong. It is not sustainable.

The high peripheral insulin levels will take any food we eat and use the food for fat storage. It might take years but at any moment of mild excess food intake above 1,000 calories, causes storage of fat don't go to build muscle or make heat it is to store fat. Survival of famine is the body's main objective.

The sponge of excess fat cells with the help of insulin will convert food to fat at low levels of calorie intake to slowly get the leptin level back to a safe level for survival. MiRNA also play a key role yet to be totally determined.

This is why you can't maintain your weight loss.

This is why your plateau usually is not even close to your optimum BMI.

Your body uses your leptin level to determine your risk of starvation.

Your reduced obese body has the same number of fat cells as your former maximum obese self and all those excess shrunken fat cells secrete an excess of MiRNA.

Your body uses the adipocytes that is has and they never go away.

If you surgically remove them, they grow back some place else.

Brain cells die. Fat cells replace themselves as they are more important for survival.

Obese individuals are Leptin resistant and often insulin resistant.

Thus Leptin and Insulin acts differently in the obese state.

They also act differently in the reduced obese state which is why people cannot maintain their weight loss despite low calorie diet and exercise.

"The answer is that there is a convergence of evidence from multiple lines of inquiry—"

Part of the anorexic pathway:

Leptin

Insulin

Ileal Brake controls rate at which food moves through the gut. It is a form of gut traffic control.

Locaserin acitvates POMC neurons in brain.

Alpha MSH release

Part of Feed stimulatory pathway

Ghrellin opposes Leptin effect in hypothalamus. Leptin inhibits ghrelin action.

Ghrelin activates NPY/AgRP neuron

Ghrelin stimulate NPY release and AgRP release increase orexigenic pathway.

The above is a short summary that is based in science and on my Obesity Boards.

Medications were designed to affect these pathways. Brain makes compensations with one medicine, thus multiple medicines needed to affect many of the different pathways.

6

TREATMENT OF CHRONIC OBESITY

My approach is for a patient to lose weight on any diet that has worked for them before. I suggest they continue the same exercise they were doing before the diet. If they injure themselves in the middle of a diet, the decrease in exercise will sabotage the program.

The diet book industry does very well because any reduction in calories will work in the 6-9 month period of weight loss before the plateau kicks in.

When does the disease of Chronic Obesity start? Dr. Aronne suggests perhaps if you have been yo-yo dieting for years? In this epidemic of Obesity I suspect if you went over a BMI of 30 and then lost 10% of your weight, you became one of the reduced obese and have billions of fat cells that are shrunken in size. This state (Sponge syndrome) constantly tells your brain your are starving because your Leptin level is low and subsequently the excess fat cells release MiRNA to cause weight regain even at low calorie level. I suspect it is the huge number of adipocytes (fat cells) that cause weight regain. I don't believe slowly increasing low glycemic foods in the reduced obese will "reprogram" the fat cells as Dr. Ludwig writes in his book, *Always Hungry.*

The solution.

1. Exercise: Walk 20 minutes a day for health, not weight loss
2. Diet: Ad libitum diet for life that does not allow you to be hungry
3. Diet medication: Once you hit the plateau and become one of the reduced obese the medications will help you maintain your weight loss and perhaps help you lose more weight.

To keep a patient on a diet medicine without clinical benefit (or 5% weight loss) is probably off label. An obesity physician should not be restricted by a rule that is not looking at individual patients who will need multiple diet medications to cover multiple pathways of weight regain.

THREE DIETS

ONE

Atkins is an ad libitum diet (this means you eat till you are full, which is difficult for the obese to stop eating even when they are full).

No calorie counting

Fat makes food taste good (butter, mayonnaise)

Protein satisfies appetite.

Easy to follow, just don't eat carbohydrates.

TWO

The first goal with the KISS diet is to keep it simple and use 4 prepared meals to calculate calories accurately.

The second goal is to put the patient in nutritional ketosis and high protein to prevent hunger. (it may not end cravings)

If you do not have positive urine strip for ketone after 2-3 weeks, I suggest you try blood strips for ketones.

If still not in ketosis, try to fast for one or two days to get into nutritional ketosis.

If you can keep carbs down to six days a week and not binge on them the Atkins might still work for you.

I know if I bring ice cream into the house or a whole pizza, I can't limit my portions.

If I don't eat high protein (30 grams or more) breakfast, lunch and dinner I get very hungry between meals. When I do get hungry between meals I eat a protein snack that has at least 10 grams of protein. Atkins French Vanilla shake is 160 cal, 2g CHO (carbs), and 15 grams protein. I also eat Almonds or Pistachios.

Even with the high protein diet, the more I exercise the more hungry I get.

I found diet medication clearly allowed me to eat less on the same Atkins diet and exercise yet still lose weight. Diet medication has also allowed me to not regain on same diet and exercise without increased hunger.

For people not able to lose weight or need a short term diet when re-gaining try the *new KISS diet:*

It's not ad libitum but when motivated this can be done for the short term.

<u>KISS(Keep It Simple Stupid) diet Calories Protein Carb</u>

1. Breakfast: 3 eggs and 3 eggs 465 27g 0g
2. Snack: Atkins vanilla shake 160 15g 2g
3. Lunch: Atkins frozen meals(Beef in Merlot) 310 20g 10g
4. Snack: Atkins vanilla shake 160 15g 2g
5. Dinner: 6-10 oz. of a meat (beef fillet 6 oz.) 414 44g 0g
6. Blue cheese dressing (2 tbsp) with salad 150 1g 1g

7. <u>Snack: Light and Lively Greek Yogurt 80 12g 9g</u>

Total 1739 calories 134g protein 24g carbohydrate
Also:

8. Stay hydrated, if cramps or feeling weak, drink Chicken bouillon for salt replacement.
9. Multivitamin
10. If constipated add low calorie metamucil

The first goal with the KISS diet is to keep it simple and use 4 prepared meals to calculate calories accurately.

The second goal is to put the patient in nutritional ketosis and high protein to prevent hunger. (it may not end cravings)

If you do not have positive urine strip for ketone after 2-3 weeks, I suggest you try blood strips for ketones.

If still not in ketosis, try to fast for one or two days to get into nutritional ketosis.

I am only suggesting this diet for short term 1-6 mos if your diet or Atkins ad libitum isn't working. Walk 20-40 minutes a day for health.

Vegan can be an ad libitum diet? I worry that high carbohydrates in insulin resistant patients is the wrong approach.

Three

The Bon Vivant diet allows you to eat till you are full. Follow Atkins diet for satiety or no hunger. It allows alcohol 1-2 oz. (some may find they lose willpower with alcohol, I found it helped decrease cravings especially after dinner for dessert).

Exercise is not strenuous. 20 minute mile walk a day is sufficient. Avoid being sedentary.

This is a substantial change but it is a change that can be done for life with help of diet medications as the medicine fights off the hunger of the decreased Leptin and increased MiRNA.

Ultimately, the treatment of the reduced obese' low level of leptin will be multiple diet medications as there are multiple hormonal pathways to prevent you from starving.

7

WHAT DOCTORS READ ABOUT LOW CARBOHYDRATE DIETS

I paid $500 to get the latest information on medical science on the internet site: UpToDate.

This is what I got for my money on Low Carbohydrate Diets.

Obesity in adults: Dietary therapy

Author

George A Bray, MD et. al.

All topics are updated (in UPTODATE) as new evidence becomes available and our peer review process is complete.

Literature review current through: Jul 2016. |

This topic last updated: Jun 15, 2016.

"Low- and very-low-carbohydrate diets are more effective for short-term weight loss than low-fat diets, although probably not for **long-term** weight loss.

A meta-analysis of five trials found that the difference in weight loss at six months, favoring the low-carbohydrate over low-fat diet, was not sustained at 12 months."

A good head to head 2 year trial is the Shai Trial. Head to head diets of low fat, Mediterranean and low carb diet were compared. LCHF did the most weight loss after two years.

8

NUTRITIONAL KETOSIS

Ketogenic diets better at weight loss?

I have presented two excellent scientific articles on Obesity (Greenway in chapter 3 and Ochner in chapter 5) where nutritional ketosis is never discussed.

In my Obesity Board training it was taught that VLCD or Very Low Calorie Diets less than 1,000 calories usually result in nutritional ketosis and this suppresses appetite.

Surprise Secret Weapon of Diets :
MEAL REPLACEMENTS

To my surprise the answer to the question, what is the most effective way to lose weight was meal replacements. I believe it is very useful to maintain weight. I eat Atkins meals as they are high in protein and low in carbs. Eating prepared meals prevents you from under estimating your daily calorie count. Using them for short terms when you have a minor weight gain might be helpful.

Simplicity is key to treatment of chronic obesity.

Fancy recipes decrease compliance.

A prepared meal with an exact amount of calories is the perfect tool for the lifelong dieter to turn to at various times in their ever changing stressful life.

My problem was my hunger would not even begin to be satisfied with one meal.

Prepared meals begin to be satisfying in VLCD (very low calorie diets) when patients are in nutritional ketosis and subsequently have their hunger blunted.

Unfortunately in the reduced obese after the plateau when the Sponge theory kicks in, nutritional ketosis and protein satiation are not enough. The low Leptin level from the shrunken fat cells will make the Reduced obese want to eat several meal replacements even though these meals are high in protein and low in carbohydrates. Imagine now the patient has been told to walk 10,000 steps a day to break through the plateau. The hunger is incredible and a meal replacement will not suffice.

However, as the Reduced obese monitor their weight every day while doing their one mile a day walk for health, if they notice a weight regain, meal replacements are a perfect way for the patient to make certain his portion size is not getting too large. It also is satisfying for hunger if the patient is also on diet medications.

Price is an issue but still cheaper than Gastric bypass surgery.

9

CAN MUSCLE BE PRESERVED WITH WEIGHT LOSS?

You can't outrun your fork but maybe with certain weight lifting programs and 2.4g/kg/d protein. The lean obese must use lean body weight.

Reynolds Article on how to gain muscle with more protein

"Exercise, particularly lifting weights, provides a signal for muscle to be retained even when you're in a big calorie deficit," says Phillips.

Researchers were intrigued because the high-protein group also lost more body fat."

I gained muscle on Atkins while in nutritional ketosis with one hour weight lifting & walking a day and extra protein from 5-3-15 weight **238** lbs to 6-23: 241.5 lbs.(weight done on home scale, no breakfast, no clothes)

My total muscle mass on my first Bioelectrical weight scale done at LA Obesity conference in Obesity Clinic Numbers

Total H2O: 49.9%

Weight:244.8 w clothes

Total body fat 31%

Fat Free mass 68.9%

Muscle Mass 46.1 lbs

6-24: started Qsymia 3.75/23 mg stopped wt lifting

I documented this with a bioelectrical impedance scale.

Second Gretchen Reynold article from NYT

This second Gretchen article suggests 3 sets of low weight lifting at 25 reps four times a week,

In my 65 year old body, I found getting to 25 repetitions quite difficult even at the lowest weight.

Elderly men develop sarcopenia mostly with muscle loss in their legs. Thus try to do leg weight lifting at the very least.

The Aronne (Zickerman) method of 2 workouts a week of 10 minutes of absolute muscle failure seem guaranteed to cause injury despite their advice to go super slow.

It's the final 10 seconds of going for the burn that worries me.

That is the injury zone in my old mind. This is more for young people.

Last month I increased my exercised by about 300%.
I doubled my walks to 40 minutes a day.
Circuit weight lifting 2-3 days a week.
Water aerobics 2-3 days a week.

	Wt.	Fat%	Muscle	H20	BMI
6-15-16	219.8	26.8%	41.3 lbs	54.1%	30.4
7-20-16	221.6	27.2	41.7 lbs	53.7%	30.7

I ate more with more exercise and gained some weight.
I gained 2 pounds weight with half pound of it as muscle.
Plan:
Lets see what happens with more protein and Gretchen's four sets of 25 reps of light weights four times a week.
How much protein for each individual?
2.4 grams of protein for each kg of lean body weight.
Difficult for people to figure lean body weight without bioelectrical impedance scale.

5-1-17:	Wt.	Fat%
	204 lbs	24.9%
	92.5 kgs	22.8 kg

Subtract 22.8 (total fat) from 92.5 (total body weight) = 69.7 (lean body weight)

Thus for me:
2.4 X 69.7= 167.08 grams of protein per day.

My diet yesterday:	Protein	Calories	Carbohydrates	Fiber:
Breakfast				
3 eggs fried in butter	18g	300	0	0
3 slices bacon	9g	165	0	0
Butter 1 TBSP		100		
Lunch:				
Atkins Beef	16g	310	g	3g
Almonds 28 nuts	6g	170	6g	3g
Atkins shake- vanilla	15g	160	2g	1g
Dinner				
Tenderloin fillet 7oz	56 g	490	0	0

Cauliflower 1 oz	0.5	14	1.1 g	
Butter 1 TBSP		100		
Pistachios I bag	5g	120	8g	2 g
Light/Lively yogurt	12g	80	9g	0
Martini Pear/Apple		355	18g	
Red wine 12 oz	12g	240	6g	
TOTALS	149g	2504 cal	59g	9g

"Total dietary fiber intake should be 25 to 30 grams a day from food, not supplements. Currently, dietary fiber intakes among adults in the United States average about 15 grams a day."UCSF Medical Center

I doubt this is important unless you are constipated."

10

EVIDENCE FOR WEIGHT LOSS MAINTENANCE WITH EXERCISE

How strong is evidence for exercise for weight loss and weight loss maintenance? Paul Maclean from Innovative Research answers this question with data I took from his slide at a conference.

to Improve Maintenance of Weight Loss showed:

Two trials said yes to benefit of exercise for weight loss maintenance

Jeffery 2003

Pavlou 1986

Eight Trials said no to exercise and weight loss maintenance

Wing 1998

Tate 2007

Skender 1996

Fogelholm 2000

Perri 1986

Leemarkers 1999

Borg 2002

Jakicic 2008

Paul MacLean, Ph.d presented the above information at Fall Obesity Summit Plenary Sessions 2015

The NLA guideline chart does not specifically address exercise advice for maintaining weight loss.

11

SPONGE SYNDROME IN THE REDUCED OBESE

Can You Eat 7 Calories/Pound a Day And Walk 5 Miles Every Day of Your Life to Maintain Your Weight?

The above formula is how the people in the National Weight Registry Program maintained their weight loss over 5 years.

The guidelines are based on the success of the reduced obese who have lost 30 lbs and maintained that weight loss over 5 years. If these 10,000 people could do it, then the rest of us should be able to do it.

However, for people with Chronic Obesity this is very difficult because of the Sponge syndrome. Who has the disease of chronic obesity? If you have lost a significant amount of weight (more than 10%) and despite your best efforts you eventually gain the weight back over 5-10 years. Some might say you have yo-yo dieting? The sponge syndrome is why this happens. A good rule might be to never get to BMI of 30, too many fat cells that never go away. 2-What is the sponge syndrome? I first wrote about The Sponge Syndrome in my book The Tubby Traveler from Topeka published in 2012. No matter how much weight you lose, the fat cells do not disappear. They shrink. Published online 5 May 2008 | Nature | doi:10.1038/news.2008.800 Fat cell numbers stay constant through adult life "Even serious weight loss doesn't reduce your overall number of fat-holding cells." Michael Hopkin "The researchers also measured 20 people who were obese and had 'stomach stapling' surgery to reduce food intake. When Spalding and her team measured these volunteers again two years after the procedure, they found no reduction in fat-cell number: the subjects still had over 80 billion individual fat cells in their bodies, Spalding and her colleagues calculate." "Nevertheless, fat cells are constantly dying and being replaced, even in adults, Spalding and her team found." These adipocytes are low in Leptin and tell your brain that you are starving. This happens before you reach your optimum BMI or body weight. Your brain is anticipating starvation before all your fat is gone. Not good for survival. The leptin starts sending messages to your brain before you have hit what you think is your ideal weight when you graduated High School or what the BMI charts suggest you should be for your height. MiRNA(packaged as episomes via blood stream) is also send out from the adipocytes out to the cells of the body to help regain weight. My Sponge theory based on low Leptin levels in lifelong cells was supported by a NEJM article published on October 27, 2011 by Priya Sumithran et al 365:1597-1604 October 27, 2011 Here is a quote from that article which I mentioned in my prior book, The Tubby Traveler from Topeka. "Worldwide, there are more than 1.5 billion overweight adults, including 400 million who are obese. Although dietary restriction often results in initial weight loss, the majority of obese dieters fail to maintain their reduced weight. Understanding the barriers to maintenance of weight loss is crucial for the prevention of relapse. Body weight is centrally regulated, with peripheral hormonal signals released from the gastrointestinal tract, pancreas, and adipose tissue integrated, primarily in the hypothalamus, to regulate food intake and energy expenditure. The number of identified peripheral modulators of appetite is expanding rapidly and includes leptin, ghrelin, cholecystokinin, peptide YY, insulin, pancreatic polypeptide, and glucagon-like peptide 1 (GLP-1).

1. Caloric restriction results in acute compensatory changes, including profound reductions in 1-energy expenditure and
2. levels of leptin and
3. cholecystokinin and
4. increases in ghrelin and appetite, all of which promote weight regain."

When Leptin is low it does not inhibit Ghrelin, thus Ghrelin is activated and increases hunger.

Leptin and Insulin share the same central feeding inhibitory and thermogenic pathways. Peripherally, Insulin is anabolic:

1. stores fat in adipose
2. stores glycogen in muscle and liver

Centrally, insulin is catabolic (as is Leptin)

1. breaks down molecules to release energy

Insulin resistance is seen in:

1. prediabetes (fasting glucose 100 or greater)
2. metabolic syndrome (waist greater than 40" causing high visceral fat)
3. diabetes mellitus type 2.

IR (insulin resistance) impairs capacity of the insulin receptor to signal the fat cell to halt triglyceride breakdown by Lipase and increases glucose uptake by glucose transport proteins. This increases release of fatty acids into central circulation and decreased uptake of glucose by fat cells.

Once again Gina Kolata brings a spotlight on the false hope of diet and exercise in her article New York Times May 5-2-16 The Biggest Loser A quote from her article below: "Researchers knew that just about anyone who deliberately loses weight — even if they start at a normal weight or even underweight — will have a slower metabolism when the diet ends. So they were not surprised to see that "The Biggest Loser" contestants had slow metabolisms when the show ended. What shocked the researchers was what happened next: As the years went by and the numbers on the scale climbed, the contestants' metabolisms did not recover. They became even slower, and the pounds kept piling on. It was as if their bodies were intensifying their effort to pull the contestants back to their original weight. Mr. Cahill was one of the worst off. As he regained more than 100 pounds, his metabolism slowed so much that, just to maintain his current weight of 295 pounds, he now has to eat 800 calories a day less than a typical man his size. Anything more turns to fat."

I found the research above to be a validation of my Sponge syndrome that the reduced obese suffer from 50 types of obesity simplified to three types:

1. Never obese
2. Reduced obese with prediabetes or metabolic syndrome or diabetes.
3. Reduced obese without high sugar or metabolic syndrome.

There are many genes that predispose to obesity but are not absolutely going to cause obesity in everyone. There are rare diseases that are clearly due to genetics: Bardet-Biedl syndrome and Prader-Willi syndrome. There are other more common diseases that can cause obesity:

1. Hypothyroidism: treat with thyroid medicine.
2. Polycystic Ovarian (PCOS): metformin has been known to help
3. Cushing's syndrome: excess steroids in body
4. Medications- some psychiatric, anti-seizure, diabetic, contraceptive, protease inhibitors, antihistamines, antihypertensives Fortunately there are usually drugs in the above classes that don't cause obesity which you can ask your physician to switch you to.

"Obesity, however, is not unique in causing WAT(White Adipose Tissue) remodeling: changes in adiposity also occur with

1. aging,
2. calorie restriction,
3. cancers, and
4. diseases such as HIV infection" (lipodystrophy)"

From the article: Methods Enzymol. 2014;537:93-122. doi: 10.1016/ B978-0-12-411619-1.00006-9.

Quantifying size and number of adipocytes in adipose tissue. Parlee SD1, Lentz SI2, Mori H1, MacDougald OA3.

LIPODYSTROPHY:

As a infectious disease specialist I have seen HIV patients with lipodystrophy. At a conference many years ago someone asked if we find what causes lipodystrophy we could use it to treat obesity? It's not a pretty way to lose weight.

"Lipodystrophy is a medical condition characterized by abnormal or degenerative conditions of the body's adipose tissue...This condition is also characterized by a lack of circulating leptin which may lead to osteosclerosis." (from Wiki)

IR (insulin resistance) impairs capacity of the insulin receptor to signal the fat cell to halt triglyceride breakdown by Lipase and increases glucose uptake by glucose transport proteins. This increases release of fatty acids into central circulation and decreased uptake of glucose by fat cells.

In obese, Insulin triggers steroidogenic factor (SF-1) which promotes food intake and perpetuates obesity. Vogt et. al. CNS Signaling Trends in Endo Metab 2013; 24(2) p76-84. "The action of Insulin on the Reward Pathway Dopaminergic is thought to contribute to development of obesity, since signaling of these higher neuronal circuits can override hypothalamic signaling. High sugar or high fat diet leads to neuronal insulin resistance and dysregulation of dopamine homeostasis and dopamine homeostasis leading to HYPODOPAMINERGIC REWARD DEFICIT SYNDROME. Wagner et la

12

SPONGE SYNDROME VALIDATION

I believe my Sponge theory as the main cause of Chronic Obesity to be verified from multiple scientific discoveries. Most important is that we do not know what has caused the epidemic of obesity in the world. Gaining weight and losing weight is relatively easy. Maintaining the weight loss is the challenge.

Guidelines advise: Maintain weight loss with more exercise and watch the calories around 1,000 to 1,500 depending on your height.

This guideline has only worked for about 5% of the chronic obese over the long term.

The Leptin hormonal theory of weight regain in the reduced obese has clearly been elucidated. The Leptin theory has also been validated by many medications that fool leptin by telling your brain it is not starving by several different hormonal pathways downstream from leptin which are on the market.

Fact: weight loss and bariatric surgery do not reduce the number of fat cells, they cause shrinkage of the adipocytes with subsequent low levels of Leptin which acts directly on the brain.

Fact: small fat cells are more efficient at gaining weight in reduced obese. There are Leptin receptors throughout the body and the adipocytes also send out MiRNA to tell the body via episomes to regain weight. Most diet books ignore all this science. As Dr. Aronne reminds us that it takes new science up to 14 years to accept the new data.

Nutrition science might be considered an oxymoron.

Nutrition science has three very good trials.

1. The Predimed trial
2. The Look Ahead trial.
3. DASH diet trial to treat hypertension.

Unfortunately we don't know if the secret sauce in the Predimed is wine and nutritionists discount the Look Ahead outcomes.

"Consilience of inductions. Call it a "convergence of evidence."
Not found for low fat diet despite multiple efforts.
Not found for exercise to maintain weight loss.

I pushed the Sponge theory as a common sense answer to why people regain their weight loss.

What the nutritionists and the guidelines push to maintain weight loss has not worked. To give the same advice to maintain weight loss that doesn't work for 80-95% of the reduced obese might be called insanity.

Resistance to low carbohydrate high fat (LCHF) has been fierce. There is finally a paradigm shift. Some studies have shown some people do better on low fat diets but overall the data for LCHF is excellent. Is it genetics or is it cultural? Shifting from high carbohydrate diet to low carbohydrate diet is a difficult change in lifestyle but it possible if you stick with the Atkins type (LCHF) long enough to get over the love of carbohydrates. I suspect the difficulty is cultural more than genetic. Time will tell. I want people to lose weight with whatever diet worked before. Once they hit the plateau of weight loss, the low fat diet fails in the long run because it is not ad libitum as the Atkins type diet is. To be able to stay on a diet for life it must satiate hunger (high protein and nutritional ketosis). Also fat gives much of food it's flavor. You need to follow a reduced calorie diet that you can stay on for the rest of your life just to maintain your weight loss, not for more weight loss.

Not matter what diet you go on, eventually it will fail because none of them reduced the number of fat cells.

Only diet medications will overcome the low Leptin levels that tell your brain the body is starving. This is science that is often not mentioned in articles on weight loss maintenance. I have tried to present some of the science without getting too much into the weeds. I have tried to keep the science as simple as possible. I took the American Board of Obesity boards. Unfortunately the other disciplines don't know or will accept this data from the Boards.

Thus "convergence of evidence" went awry during the decades of low fat dieting. Possibly the influence of the food production lobbyists had something to do with it. Dr. Ludwig writes about guidelines allowing fruit juices might have to do with lobby interests on the guideline board in his tweets. "Satisfying America's Fruit Gap: Summary of an Expert Roundtable on the Role of 100% Fruit Juice First published: 6 June 2017 Abstract:

"The 2015 to 2020 Dietary Guidelines for Americans (DGAs) recognize the role of 100% fruit juice in health and in helping people meet daily fruit recommendations and state that 100% fruit juice is a nutrient-dense beverage that should be a primary choice, along with water and low-fat/fat-free milk."

For my Sponge syndrome "to overturn the consensus, I would need to find flaws with all the lines of supportive evidence and show a consistent convergence of evidence toward a different theory that explains the data."

The Hall analysis of the Biggest Loser puts a big question mark next to the advice of exercise and low calorie intake as that did not work for 13 of 15 people in the trial.

The Look Ahead data showed that after 10 years of the best exercise and diet program with close personal support to keep behavioral changes failed in primary outcomes compared to control. This was a random controlled trial with large numbers of participants and a good control over 10 years. It doesn't get much better than this in nutrition science. Yet this data does not change the guidelines. Most guidelines still advise 90 minutes or more of exercise to maintain weight.

The key to maintaining weight loss is a low calorie diet that you can stay on the rest of your life. The answer is an ad libitum diet and diet medications.

No guidelines should be written without a close examination of the many hormonal ways the brain uses to make you gain weight again. The Sponge Syndrome is the perfect storm for weight regain in the reduced obese. The number of fat cells has the last word. I asked Dr. Leibel if adipocytes only live 10 years. He said there is some discussion of that but there is evidence that the fat cells that die are rapidly replaced. Thus the billions of excess fat cells of the obese are present for life in the reduced obese that act like a sponge for free fatty acids.

I had the privilege today of listening to Dr. Michael Rosenbaum talk about why weight loss maintenance is so difficult. I asked Dr. Rosenbaum if what I call the Sponge Syndrome might also make it difficult to maintain weight loss. Small fat cells are efficient at re-gaining fat. Since the reduced obese continued to have a large number of fat cells despite weight loss all these cells make it easy to gain weight. He asked why the skinny people with skinny fat cells don't also regain weight. I said the insulin resistance causes high levels of insulin which has abnormal increase in the dyslipidemic effects causing the fat cells to take up FFA. Also Dr. Liebel has taught about leptin thresholds changing with obesity.

Similar to the Frank Greenway review mentioned above, I was greatly gratified to find this Ochner review that also supported much of my Sponge Theory and it's cause of the Chronic Disease of Obesity

Ochner et al article Feb 11, 2015

"Irrespective of starting weight, caloric restriction triggers several biological adaptations designed to prevent starvation.[3]

These adaptations might be potent enough to undermine the long-term effectiveness of lifestyle modification in most individuals with obesity, particularly in an environment that promotes energy overconsumption."

Ochner adds **preadipocyte proliferation** *increases fat storage capacity. This goes along with what I hypothesized in my Sponge Theory.*

*Ochner also says "**that these biological adaptations often persist indefinitely**, even when a person re-attains a healthy BMI via behaviourally induced weight loss.[3]"*

In accord with the thesis of my book, The Chronic Disease of Obestiy, Ochner goes on to say "few individuals ever truly recover from obesity; individuals who formerly had obesity but are able to re-attain a healthy body weight via diet and exercise still have 'obesity in remission'

13

LOOK AHEAD

THE BIGGEST FAILURE OF DIET AND EXERCISE

This was a negative outcome trial of the best diet and exercise could do against a control group over 10 years.

Here is the data every weight loss diet book should present.
It is the best that a 10 year diet and exercise program could produce.
A 2.5% weight loss compared to control.

After 10 years of work and suffering a 2.5% improvement over the control is the best that can be achieved?
Look AHEAD had the usual waterfall weight loss results of all diet trials.

The waterfall effect of the treated group in Look AHEAD:
39.3% did maintain >10% weight loss and that is great.
However, 17.2% of the control group had > 10% weight loss after 8 years.
Remember, half of the people in the National Weight Control Registry maintain their weight loss on their own.
A great deal of money was spent over 10 years to council the treatment group with little effect and a negative trial outcome.

Quote from the NEJM paper:
"Weight loss was greater in the intervention group than the control group throughout (8.6% vs. 0.7% at 1 year;
6.0% vs. 3.5% at study end)." (2.5% difference)

False Hope of Surgery below:

It's all about adaptive thermogenesis. The shrunken fat cells don't disappear. The low Leptin level eventually causes the body to regain weight. 30% of bariatric surgery patients regain all their weight after 10 years.

Even gastric bypass surgery have waterfall results, with many patients gaining weight comparing 2 year results with 6 year results.

JAMA 2012.303(11)1122-1131

In Sponge syndrome with billions of shrunken fat cells causing weight regain after 6-9 months of weight loss because of Leptin deficiency.

This low level of Leptin cannot be treated with one maneuver.

14

BIOELECTRICAL IMPEDANCE SCALE

I had my body fat determined by calibers on skin fat on 3/27/1997. I was 45 years old
45 inch waist and
242 lbs.
My computed body fat was 27%.
I had 65 lbs of fat and my lean body weight was calculated at 177.

I think this under calculated my body fat%.
Perhaps I had much more muscle mass but calibur test did not measure that.
At age 47 I tried to join the reserves.
They did not use calibers.
Weight 240.
Waist 48 inches
Neck circumference 17.5 inches.
Determine abdominal-neck factor. 113.49
Height factor 80.25
Subtract height factor from abdominal-neck factor = 33.24% fat.
Again muscle mass not determined.
I failed my test to be a soldier. I was told 26% body fat was the maximum to get in. In this case obesity probably saved my life.
I had my first body composition with BIA scale done at Stormont Obesity Clinic on 6-25-15 at 63 years old
244.8 lbs,
Waist 43"
Total body fat 31%, 75.2 lbs.
muscle mass 46.1 lbs. But Ohms 486 was low which means muscle mass may be higher.
Fat free mass 68.9% with 167.4 lbs. This may be the lean body weight.
At age 65 I may have developed *sarcopenia*. As people age their BMI may not change but the skeletal muscle mass becomes less as more fat is put on. For men this is especially true in the legs.
Lean body weight becomes important in the Obese to determine doses of medicines. I

suspect it is rarely used for this. Need to determine lean body weight to know how many grams of protein a day to eat (2.4 mg/kg lean body weight).

BIOELECTRICAL IMPEDANCE ANALYSIS

"BIA is considered reasonably accurate for measuring groups, *or for tracking body composition in an individual over a period of time,* but is not considered sufficiently accurate for recording of single measurements of individuals."

"Two-electrode foot-to-foot measurement is less accurate than 4-electrode (feet, hands) and eight-electrode measurement."

I AM ON 5 DIET MEDICATIONS!

I recently (3-17-17) increased my liraglutide to 3.0 mg a day. This helped me get down to 200 lbs without changing my diet and only walking 20 to 40 minutes a day.

However, I lost 40 lbs since I started Invokana and stopped Insulin and Actos.

Now the challenge is to maintain weight lose in the reduced obese state as demonstrated in *THE BIGGEST LOSER by Gina Kolata*

Yesterday when I went to my Obesity Clinic at Stormont, the Nurse Practitioner who takes care of me was pleased with my body composition results.

Compare 5-16-16 when I weighed in at my lowest at 217.3 lbs to 8-17-16 at 222.5 lbs.

Without the benefit of Bioelectric Impedance Scale, one might say the five diet medications are failing.

However, in the last two months I began a high protein (2.4 mg/kg lean body weight) and circuit weight lifting of 25 repetitions to preserve muscle mass.(How to preserve muscle while losing weight)

My muscle mass increased by 1.8 lbs.
My body fat decreased by 1.1%.
My fat free mass increased by 1.2%
My body water increased by 1.6%

I did this with an AD LIBITUM ATKINS DIET. I am never hungry and I drink 2-4 oz ETOH almost everyday.

This is the Bon Vivant diet.

15

BARIATRIC SURGERY, THE LAST RESORT

I went to a conference on Obesity in Washington DC in October 2015. Dr. Denis Halmi gave a lecture titled Recidivism after Bariatric Surgery.

The most important fact I took away from that lecture on Bariatric surgery was:

"30% of patients regain the lost weight by 10 years"

I believe all diet medications should be tried before bariatric surgery is done.

Main reason is from MedlinePlus June 6, 2017

"One in Five Weight loss surgery patients using opioids." 7 years after the surgery.

To my surprise new Data from Duke in JAMA Surgery 31, 2016 Maciejewski et al. claimed

"Only 19 of 564 patients undergoing RYGB (3.4%) regained weight back to within an estimated 5% of their baseline weight by 10 years."

I looked at the data more carefully and found:

The study did 1787 RYGB surgeries. Only 19 of 564 surgical patients gained most of their weight back after 10 years. However the study did 1787 RYGB surgeries.

<u>What happened to the other 1223 patients that had surgery?</u> 68% of patients were lost to follow up?

They probably didn't go back to follow up because they gained their weight back.

If *intention to treat analysis* is done, the regain number would be much higher. This is the VA, there must be follow up data on these surgeries?

More data from the Duke study:

"Patients undergoing RYGB **lost 21%** (95% CI, 11%-31%) more of their baseline weight **at 10 years** than nonsurgical matches.

A total of 405 of 564 patients undergoing RYGB (71.8%) had more than 20% estimated weight loss, and 224 of 564 (39.7%) had more than 30% estimated weight loss at 10 years compared with *134 of 1247 (10.8%) and 48 of 1247 (3.9%), respectively, of* nonsurgical matches.

The usual waterfall results of weight loss studies:

<u>Non-surgical patients</u>

10.8% had more than 20% weight loss?

3.4% had more than 30% weight loss?

After 15 years there was data of sustained weight loss. Again the dropout rate is large and again no explanation

NYT Sept 10, 2016 Sunday Review Opinion

Dr. Sarah Hallberg and Osama Hamdy write:

"It is nonsensical that we're expected to prescribe these (bariatric) techniques to our patients while the medical guidelines don't include another better, safer and far cheaper method: a diet low in carbohydrates."

16

THE FIRST OFFICE VISIT NEEDS DATA

Concentrate on preventing arterial plaque and getting type 2 diabetes mellitus patients off Insulin and actos.

OBESITY COMORBIDITIES:

1. Type 2 diabetes mellitus
2. Hypertension
3. Hyperlipidemia
4. Cancer
5. Osteoarthritis
6. Cardiovascular disease
7. Obstructive sleep apnea
8. Asthma

If you have these conditions as a result of obesity, the risks vs. benefits of diet medications becomes apparent.

Unfortunately it is more popular to go to Bariatric surgery.

First rule, stop medicines that make you fat.

Second rule, determine if you have metabolic syndrome.

Medicines to ask your Doctor if you can replace it with some other drug.

Insulin replace with Invokana, metformin and victoza.

Much of the literature states most people cannot stay on an Atkins type diet. Stopping carbohydrates is too restrictive. I might believe that may be true in patients who are not pre-diabetic or with metabolic syndrome. When I first went on Atkins many years ago for one month. I had the weakness often associated with it. Even now I get leg cramps at bedtime. The solution for this is chicken bouillon, magnesium and perhaps potassium replacement and increased fluid intake.

All diets are restrictive. I suspect failure to give up carbohydrates is more a result of cultural and ethnic conditioning rather than genetics.

There are no essential carbohydrates. There are essential fats and amino acids. Usually after a month, less carbs can be acceptable by most people. No matter which diet the reduced obese choose they all have restrictions and must have a reduction in calories just to maintain the weight loss.

There is a carb nite that is suggested in LCHF, as long as it is not a whole pizza pie, a whole pint of ice cream or a pound of pasta. I have found the main benefit of diet medications is that they help me reduce portions and reduce hunger. I have found I have been able to skip my mid-morning snack and mid-afternoon snack if I had 30 g protein for breakfast and 30 g protein for lunch. If I need a snack I stick to a bag of pistachios 1.5 oz. (42 g) After dinner boredom or hungry is relieved by a cocktail and a Lite and Lively 80 calories Greek Yogurt cup.

I ask patients to come to the office fasting and obtain fasting glucose and fasting ketone level.

If the fasting glucose level is 100 or more then the patient has the first criteria of the Metabolic syndrome.

At this point the patient needs to start Metformin 500 mg a day.
This is possibly the first obesity drug.

One quarter of the USA population has Metabolic syndrome.
Pg 12 Current Medical Diagnosis and Treatment 2017
<u>Metabolic syndrome is defined as:</u>
Three or more of the following:

1. fasting glucose greater than 110
2. triglycerides greater than 150
3. hypertension
4. HDLc less than 40 for men and less than 50 for women
5. abdominal obesity

<u>I use the NCEP ATP 3 criteria from 2005 to diagnose Metabolic syndrome.</u>
The main difference is the fasting glucose is 100 or greater.
The measurement of the waist is done at the level of the iliac crest:

>40" or 102 cm for men
>35" or 88 cm for women
For Asians:
>89 cm for men
> 79 for women

I also will look at the triglyceride/HDLc ratio. If it is 3:1 or greater I will consider the patient has metabolic syndrome.

IR (insulin resistance) impairs capacity of the insulin receptor to signal the fat cell to halt triglyceride breakdown by Lipase and increases glucose uptake by glucose transport proteins. This increases release of fatty acids into central circulation and decreased uptake of glucose by fat cells.

I advise patients to use the diet that worked for them before. Someone who does not have pre-diabetes or metabolic syndrome or type 2 diabetes mellitus a low carb diet may not work as well for them. I would still suggest these patients switch to a low carb diet when they hit the plateau to go into nutritional ketoacidosis which may help with the low leptin causing increased hunger.

Eating ad libitum will help prevent hunger. Eat 5 times a day with high protein. Despite this change I believe the sponge syndrome overcomes this to help the patient gain weight. That is the time for diet medications to maintain weight loss. If already on diet meds, consider adding another diet medication if you continue to gain weight.

PART TWO

THE TUBBY THEORY AND CARDIOVASCULAR DISEASE

17

RISK FOR HEART ATTACK

Next step in the office visit is to determine the risk for a cardiovascular event (strokes or heart attacks).

This is done with:

Pooled Cohort Risk Assessment Equations

Predicts 10-year risk for a first atherosclerotic cardiovascular disease (ASCVD) event

My total cholesterol is too low for this calculator.

It is 119. I was forced to use a higher number is get a evaluation.

The red bar probably represents me as my blood pressure is treated and my glucose Hg A1C usually 7.0 or lower.

I advise patients to get more data.

Find out if you have atherosclerotic plaque. This will change your risk up or down.

Get a CAC (coronary artery calcium) CT calcium score($50 cash)

and a CIMT (carotid intimal media thickness) ultrasound ($100 cash)

If you have plaque or atheroma then you have the disease of atherosclerosis and it increases your risk of an event.

If your CAC is zero it decreases your risk considerably.

If you are <u>symptomatic</u> and your CAC is zero you still have a 16% risk.

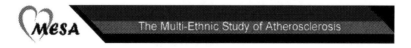

MESA 10-Year CHD Risk with Coronary Artery Calcification

The blue line says:

"The estimated 10 year risk of a CHD event for a person with this risk factor profile including coronary calcium is **12.5%**

The estimated 10 year risk of a CHD event for a person with this risk factor profile if we did factor in their coronary calcium score would be **11.1%**

Calcium score 144   Calcium volume 126

CAC is not advised on a routine follow up basis as statin treatment will cause an increase in the CAC number.

18

CIMT AND CAC

HIGH FAT DIET DID NOT EQUAL "CLOGGED ARTERIES"

Does a diet that is 60% fat (including so called bad and good fats) cause atherosclerosis? That is the big question about Atkins diet.

I documented my CIMT from 2009 till 2017 while on an Atkins diet, my results were very good.

CIMT's at KUMC in Dr. Moriarty's Lipo-apheresis clinic:

	Average CCA Mean	Average CCA Max Region
12-17-09	0.599 mm	0.741 mm
12-8-11	0.563 mm (less)	0.661 mm *(less)*
12-20-12	0.566 mm (more)	0.676 mm (more)
12-19-13	0.583 mm (more)	0.709 mm (more)
11-20-14	0.575 mm (less)	0.679 mm (less)
12-03-15	0.555 mm (less)	0.675 mm (less)
12-08-16	0.611 mm (more)	0.74 mm (more)
12-14-17	0.570 mm (less)	0.671 mm (less)

CAC reports below over 10 years:

	Calcium score	Calcium volume
2-6-01	8.93	8.02
1-10-06	20.5	57.5
12-9-11	7.9	5.9
7-21-16	144	126

Over 8 years, I have had regression.

More importantly, I have not had the progression that a age 66 year old diabetic type 2 might be expected to have over 8 years on a Atkins diet with 60% fat.

There will be natural thickening of the intimal wall with aging as well.

My CAC increased from 7.9 to 144 but this is a well known phenomenon that occurs when intensive statin therapy is used.

A good reason not to bother with follow up CAC scans too often.

I received a critique from another Fellow of the National Lipid association. I told him a 0.034 mm change in carotid wall thickness is significant from the Neil Stone Lipid manual.

My friend wrote Thomas Barringer, a national expert on CIMT or cIMT.

In summary Dr. Barringer's letter stated the following:

1. He agreed with everything my friend critiqued me about,
2. IMT "progression" has shown not association with subsequent cardiovascular events (CVE) except for,
3. The IMPROVE study (Baldassare, et al) did publish results in 2013 in which they showed that an entirely new IMT variable – *the IMT segment showing the fastest increase in maximum dimension* – was associated with an increase in CVEs.

Dr. Barringer actually validated me for my purposes.

I do not do these CIMT's for determining cardiovascular risk.

My purpose was to determine if I would lay on substantial plaque in carotids due to being on a Atkins 60% fat diet. Most of the fat was beef, eggs, bacon, butter and mayonnaise. Not the so called "good" fats of the Mediterranean diet.

19

WHAT IS THE BEST CHOLESTEROL TEST?

LDLp vs LDLc vs non-HDLc vs. Remnants

In my opinion I think it is the Liposcience LDLp done by Nuclear magnetic resonance.
The second best is the non-HDL cholesterol test because it is the cheapest.
The third is the apoB test.

The new view is to determine the number of cholesterol remnants on your lab test. The formula is to subtract LDLc and HDLc from Total cholesterol. The result is the amount of cholesterol remnants.

For example:
My total cholesterol was 115
Subtract LDLc -57
Total *58*
Subtract HDLc -48
Total cholesterol remnants 10 (greater than 30 is high?)

Patients need to have their Doctors change from following a patient's LDLc to non-HDLc at the very least. There is too much discordance between LDLc and LDLp especially in patients with Metabolic syndrome, Diabetes Mellitus or high triglyceride level.

Wednesday, January 13, 2016

Official guidelines for LDLp and apoB seem a little high to me

In my book *The Tubby Theory from Topeka* written at the end of 2009, I advised that non-HDL-C be called the Tubby Factor as it is easier to remember to ask your Doctor, what is my Tubby Factor?
Non-HDL-C is more accurate in predicting future risk than the LDL-C.

More accurate than both of those is the particle number
(don't get bogged down with particle size, HDLc or Triglycerides).
ApoB and LDLp are the best tests.
LDLp Ion method done by Quest lab does not use the numbers in this chart.
The apoB by Quest is the same range as this chart.

AACE lipid targets for Patients with Type 2 Diabetes and one major ASCVD risk factor or established ASCVD:

LDLc <70
non-HDL <100
Triglycerides < 150
Apo B (particles) < 80
LDLp (particles) <1,000

Major risk factors include:

1. family history of ASCVD,
2. high blood pressure,
3. low HDLc,
4. smoking.

Executive summary, Endocrine Practices 2016;22(No.1)

ACC publishes consensus document on non-statin therapies for LDL reduction
April 2, 2016

One way to know if you have atherosclerotic disease is to get a CAC and CIMT. Guidelines do advise using these studies for further clarification of risk.

With the publication of studies such as IMPROVE-IT and HPS2-THRIVE. The cholesterol guideline states that non-statin therapies may be considered in patients who respond poorly to statins or cannot tolerate optimal doses of them.

"Non-statin options
If it is decided that a non-statin therapy should be pursued, options to consider include

1. referral to a lipid specialist and
2. registered dietitian nutritionist,
3. ezetimibe (Zetia, Merck),
4. bile acid sequestrants and
5. PCSK9 inhibitors such as alirocumab (Praluent, Sanofi/Regeneron) and evolocumab (Repatha, Amgen). Mipomersen (Kynamro, Isis Pharmaceutical/Genzyme), lomitapide (Juxtapid, Aegerion) and

6. LDL apheresis may be considered by lipid specialists for <u>patients with familial hypercholesterolemia</u>, Lloyd-Jones and colleagues wrote."

References:

Lloyd-Jones DM. Dyslipidemia Combo-Therapy: A Framework for Clinical Decision-Making. Presented at: American College of Cardiology Scientific Session; April 2-4, 2016; Chicago.

<u>Lloyd-Jones DM, et al. *J Am Coll Cardiol.* 2016;doi:10.1016/j.jacc.2016.03.519.</u>

It is outrageous that Niacin removed from the non-statin therapy.

This removal of niacin is based on an inaccurate analysis of IMPROVE-IT and HPS2-THRIVE.

One of the best Lipidologist writes how he approaches the problem of treatment with statins and non-statins:

"Dr Sniderman: The first thing I do is measure apoB to determine whether treatment is necessary or not.

<u>If apoB is elevated, then all things being equal, treatment needs to be seriously considered.</u> Treatment is a collaborative process between the patient and the physician and involves diet, exercise, and lifestyle as well as pharmacologic agents if indicated.

For the majority, my target for LDL-lowering therapy is an apoB < 75 mg/dL.

For those at very high risk, my target is an apoB < 65 mg/dL.

These are the equivalent population levels to the LDL-C and non–HDL-C targets chosen by many recent guideline groups. The apoB targets chosen by many of the guideline groups are much too high. It seems that once 1 group selected values, the others just repeated them."

<u>Above quote from Lipid Round table article</u>

Thus according to this last CIMT I have not had regression but I also have not had the progression at age 65 diabetic type 2 that might be expected over 7 years. There will be natural thickening of the intimal wall with aging

Likewise my CAC increased from 7.9 to 144 but this is a well known phenomenon that occurs when intensive statin therapy is used. A good reason not to bother with follow up CAC scans.

In high risk patients I try to get the following goals(in my book from 2009):

1. Tubby Factor (Non-HDLc)less than 80. INEXPENSIVE TEST
2. LDLc less than 70 USUALLY CALCULATED AND INACCURATE IN INSULIN RESISTANCE
3. apo B less than 60 (immunoassay) PARTICLE COUNT
4. LDLp less than 750 (done by Liposcience NMR) PARTICLE COUNT- BEST TEST MY OPINION

The 2014 American Diabetic guidelines are still using the old LDLc.

Diabetics often have discordance between LDLc and Tubby Factor and Particle number.

The National Lipid Association now uses non-HDL cholesterol as an official target. I predicted this in my book in 2009. LDLp and apoB still not an official target of any group.

Contrary to the ACC/AHA guidelines, the NLA guidelines state non-statin therapy should be considered in patients who can't tolerate statin therapy or high dose statin therapy. Non-Statin therapy medicines by a second or third agent may be considered for patients who have not reached goals for atherogenic cholesterol levels.

20

TUBBY THEORY FROM TOPEKA UPDATE

My book, _The Tubby Theory from Topeka_ published Jan 2010 p. 9:

"The _Tubby Theory_ is that we can prevent heart disease with simvastatin/Endur-acin in America for less than $100 a year if we find the subclinical atherosclerosis _early_ with CAC/CIMT." I wrote this in Dec. 2009.

Cardiologists did not know what a non-HDL cholesterol was? _The ignored number_ in Tim Russert's(anchor on Meet the Press NBC) life and his post mortem analysis was his non-HDL cholesterol.

Apparently no one asked a lipidologist?

Subtract HDLc from total cholesterol = non-HDL cholesterol. (or Tubby Factor)

Last month I learned that remnant particles should be calculated as well.

Remnant cholesterol = Total cholesterol

Minus HDLc

<u>Minus LDLc</u>

= Remnant cholesterol

Today in 2017 I will update Tim Russert's risk not recognized by me before:

Total cholesterol 155

Minus LDLc 68

Minus HDLc 37

Equals 50

The remnants are abnormally high.

I think the Tubby Theory has held up well, as demonstrated below. Many experts now believe (Robinson and Allan Sniderman) treating early will improve outcomes. CAC and CIMT are tools to convince the patient to start statins early in a non-symptomatic patient. However, the mistake to go to high dose statin in many cases.

I advised

1. lowest statin dose

    Check non-HDLc if not at goal don't increase statin, take

2. Enduracin 1,000mg(over the counter niacin with proprietary wax matrix formula) Check non-HDL and if not at goal take don't increase dose to avoid side effects. Instead take

3. Ezetimibe (Zetia) sometimes one half a tablet is sufficient.

To support this approach

Update on Tubby Theory from Topeka 2008 to 2016
<u>8 years later</u>
<u>A friend asks me:</u>

<u>"You have been talking about Coronary Calcium Score for a long time. Were you ahead of your colleagues, or in step?</u>

I wrote the book The Tubby Theory from Topeka after I passed the lipid boards and Tim Russert died.
No one in NLA spoke on National media that Russert's non-HDLc was not treated to goal.

I guess they were afraid of being sued.
I thus wrote a book about treating patients in my practice aggressively.
I used the teachings of my mentors at NLA.
I quote them (my mentors) throughout my book.

My only originality was to call non-HDLc the Tubby Factor because patients and physicians could not remember "non-HDL cholesterol" nor how to calculate it.
I called it the Tubby factor because non-HDLc is usually discordant with LDLc in patients with metabolic syndrome. ⅘ of these patients are Obese usually with central obesity.
Since my book in 2008 I have been gratified to see that CAC and CIMT have proven themselves as significant and independent risk predictors for CVD.
New AHA/ACA guidelines in 2013 by Stone use CAC or CIMT in low risk patients to determine if statins should be started or not.
Niacin is under attack as being a dangerous drug which I believe is just silly. If low dose *wax matrix niacin (over the counter Endur-acin)* 1,000 mg/d is used with low dose lipitor 20 mg/d early in the disease of subclinical atherosclerosis for long term treatment I believe we can prevent most CVD. Some patients will need Zetia (now available in generic form ezetimibe.)
I am very proud of my book, *The Tubby Theory from Topeka,* and still stand by it.
Even the low fat diet I suggested might be suitable for some folks who are insulin sensitive and hyper-absorbers of cholesterol. Atkins doesn't work for everyone. In the present obesity epidemic I think most obese have pre-diabetes or metabolic syndrome. Atkin's type diet is the best for these people. My experience with being on a 60% fat Atkins diet since 2011 did not increase my atheroma on CIMT or CAC People should use the diet that worked for them before. Ultimately for life-long maintenance of weight loss I advise switching to Atkins as you

can eat ad libitum and test yourself for nutritional ketosis. Most reduced obese will ultimately need diet medicines to not feel the terrible hunger that low leptin will cause after years of dieting.

There was an article by Denise Grady (see reference 7) about Tim Russert's death.

My opinion about Ms. Grady's article:
Yes we could pinpoint the higher risk at that time.
Mr. Russert needed to have his non-HDL cholesterol calculated.
Total cholesterol minus HDLc. These two articles never mention this.
The NYT does not mention Glagov remodeling of the arteries which is why a nuclear stress test was false negative in Mr Russert one month before his death.
To my knowledge I am the only one who wrote about this in 2009 in my book.
A CIMT would have alerted the physician that Mr Russert's carotid artery was thick with plaque.

In the metabolic patient such as Mr Russert there is usually discordance between LDLc and LDLp or non-HDLc.
Mr Russert was thought to have normal LDLc. With his high triglycerides this is very unlikely.
Once a simple test of subtraction was done and the Non-HDLc was found to not be at normal, the LDLp or apo B particle test should have been done.
Then those numbers could have been treated to goal by more medicine.

In my book 2009, I advise my patients get the
LDLp < 750
Apo B < 60
non-HDL cholesterol < 80
If they have plaque on their CAC or CIMT to reverse that plaque.

In May 2008 Tim Russert's non-HDL cholesterol was 118 (TC 155- HDLC 37)
He was clearly not treated to goal with the information at hand.
There is even discordance with non-HDLc and particle number. A $100 blood test for particle number should also be obtained before an $1,000 invasive angiogram is obtained.
Some doctors say people like Mr. Russert, with no symptoms but risk factors like a thickened heart, **should have angiograms,** in which a catheter is threaded into the coronary arteries, dye is injected, and X-rays are taken to look for blockages.
Again this is a picture of the lumen of the artery.
Very likely, most of Mr. Russert's disease *was in the wall of the artery* only to be seen by IVUS (intravascular ultrasound).
However CIMT could give a guess as to what might be going on in the wall of the coronary

artery if the thickness of the carotid wall was much thicker than it should be. In my practice, I had 11 patients with negative CAC but positive CIMT. They complement each other.

The NYT article by Denise Grady also says statins only reduce risk by 70%, leaving a residual risk of 30%.

My response:

The Multiplier effect is to treat the other residual risk of 30%.

Find the plaque early with CAC and CIMT.

Treat early and for a long period with low dose combination therapy.

Low dose to avoid side effects the long term.

Keep LDLp < 750 or 1,000.

This is what I said in the Tubby Theory in 2009.

I showed the results of doing it in my practice in my book.

I wrote the Tubby Theory of Topeka to alert people that the sudden surprise death of Tim Russert could have been prevented if the discordance between LDLc and non HDL-cholesterol had been recognized. Better data with LDL particle number should have been done. Now with PCSK9 we know LDLc levels of 39 mg/dl are therapeutic and reduce plaque as determined by IVUS (Intravascular Ultrasound.)

GLAGOV TRIAL

Nov. 15,2016

Global Assessment of Plaque Regression With a PCSK9 Antibody as Measured by Intravascular Ultrasound - GLAGOV

Nov 15, 2016 'Interpretation:

Among patients with angiographic evidence of coronary artery disease and on chronic statin therapy, the PCSK9 inhibitor evolocumab resulted in a greater change in percent atheroma volume and a greater proportion of patients with plaque regression. Although not powered for clinical outcomes, major adverse cardiac events were numerically reduced with evolocumab. Larger studies powered for clinical outcomes are warranted."

21

NIACIN STILL A GREAT DRUG

GUIDELINES CHOOSE DRUGS WITHOUT HEAD TO HEAD TRIALS?

"In the absence of **high quality head-to-head drug comparison trials** to determine the relative efficacy of the individual drugs, choice of therapy should be based upon

1. efficacy,
2. safety,
3. *cost*,
4. convenience,
5. and other patient-related factors."

The above is from *Up To Date* on choosing drugs for *Osteoporosis*.

Consensus Committee April 6, 2016

ACC Expert Consensus Decision Pathway on the Role of Non-Statin Therapies for LDL-Cholesterol Lowering in the Management of Atherosclerotic Cardiovascular Disease Risk.
"the value of patient-provider interaction in clinical decision making when *non-statin* therapies are considered,

1. examining the extent of available scientific evidence for net clinical benefit,
2. safety and
3. tolerability,
4. potential for drug-drug interactions,
5. *efficacy of additional LDL-C lowering,*
6. *cost,*
7. convenience and
8. medication storage,
9. pill burden,
10. route of administration, and
11. patient preference"

<u>NEJM article Head to Head trial:</u>
<u>Niacin vs. Zetia (ezetimibe)</u>
N Engl J Med 2009; 361:2113-2122

"As compared with ezetimibe, niacin had greater efficacy regarding the change in mean carotid intima–media thickness over 14 months (P=0.003), leading to significant reduction of both mean (P=0.001) and maximal carotid intima–media thickness

Paradoxically, greater reductions in the LDL cholesterol level in association with ezetimibe were significantly associated with an increase in the carotid intima–media thickness Interestingly there are **head to head trials** with Niacin."

Most famous is the <u>Coronary Drug Project </u>in which "Mortality in the niacin group was 11% lower than in the placebo group (52.0 versus 58.2%; p = 0.0004)" after 15 years. Not a blinded random control study.

Yet somehow Niacin failed to make the list of non-statin drugs allowed on the list yet PCSK9 which is $1,000 a month, has one outcome study and is given intravenously is on the list?

Reference from Table 26.2 from J.R. Guyton et. al.

List of Randomized niacin trials with clinical cardiovascular outcomes:

1. HATS: Clinical events reduced by 70%
2. AFREGS: Clinical events reduced by 50%
3. CLAS: more overall regression of plaque (p<0.002)
4. UCSF-SCOR: Coronary angio regression (p<0.039)
5. FATS: regression of plaque and 73% reduced clinical events (P<0.05)
6. HARP: no change in coronary angiographic progression.
7. ARBITER 2-3: Mean regression of CIMT at 2 years (p< 0.001)
8. THOENES CIMT: Mean regression of CIMT (p=0.021)
9. ARBITER-6 HALTS: Reduction CIMT (p <0.001)
10. CAROTID MRI: Reduction in carotid wall area by MRI (p=0.03)

Niacin was dropped from guidelines because AIM-HIGH and HPS-THRIVE were stopped early.

These were not LDLc lowering trials. LDLc was already at goal with statins.
These were HDLc and triglyceride trials.
The guidelines don't have targets for HDLc and advise triglycerides less than 500. The major goal is to lower LDLc. Niacin lowers LDLc even after year three of the AIM HIGH trial.
Why then, was Niacin dropped from guidelines?
5-"efficacy of additional LDL-C lowering,"

IMPROVE-IT TRIAL with Zetia.

"It took 7 years of follow-up for us to reach that many events, so some investigators were wondering if this would be the eternal trial," Cannon said. "But that was really good news because it meant that the treatment was working: we were actually doing good for our patients."

It should, however, be noted that 42% of patients, regardless of treatment, stopped the study drug before the end of the trial.

Zetia was added to the list by the consensus committee because it had the IMPROVE-IT positive outcome.

If AIM-HIGH went out to 7 years it may also have had a positive outcome for Niacin. It was a government study however.

There were some illnesses in patients on Niacin and AIM-HIGH was stopped early. Later these illnesses were found not to be statistically significant but I believe it is the reason the committee left Niacin off the list of advised drugs.

At the Philadelphia NLA meeting in May 20, 2017, several speakers said they don't use Niacin anymore because of "toxic" side effects from Niacin in AIM HIGH and HPS- THRIVE.

However there are other opinions:

"Recent results published by the two large clinical studies, AIM-HIGH and HPS-THRIVE, have led to the impugnation of niacin's role in future clinical practice. However, due to several methodological flaws in the AIM-HIGH and HPS2-THRIVE studies, the pleiotrophic effects of niacin now deserve thorough evaluation."

ACTA PHARM
2016 DEC 1;66(4): 449-469 Zeman M et. al.

Last year at the NLA master's program the slide bullet stated:

"Significant excesses of serious adverse events (SAEs) due to known and unrecognized side-effects of niacin. Over 4 years, ER niacin/laropiprant caused SAEs in approximately 30 patients per 1,000."

Specifically in HPS2-THRIVE:
Coronary death Placebo had 0.1% less 302 vs 291 p 0.63
Hemorrhagic stroke Placebo had 0.2% less 114 vs. 89 p 0.08
These are not significant differences.
"If the p-value is less than **0.05**, we reject the null hypothesis that there's no difference between the means and conclude that a significant difference does exist."

Slide on effect of ERN/LRPT on serious adverse events with significant p:
Diabetic complication 3.7%
New onset diabetes 1.8%
Infection 1.4%
Gastrointestinal 1.0%

The problem with these SAEs with a significant p is we don't know if niacin is responsible or LRPT.

What I find difficult to understand is why Niacin's legacy effect has been ignored. It has decades of efficacy and safety and is inexpensive. PCSK9 is expensive but can get LDLc down to 39. Patients at high risk who can't take statins need this. The Tubby Theory alternative is to take the lowest dose of a statin plus Enduracin(over the counter niacin) 1,000 mg plus zetia. This combination needs to be attempted before using the very expensive PCSK9 drug. The lower doses have less side effects and the three drugs are very likely to get to goal as I showed in my list of patients in my book from 2010.

Since I wrote Tubby Theory from Topeka the data has confirmed the premise that the lower the LDLc the better.

Thus most believe it is not the pleiotrophic effects or the raising of HDLc that improve treatment, it is how low can you get the patient's LDLc down. (beware of discordance between LDLc, nonHDL-c and LDLp and apoB)

Many might believe the pill burden to be too great. Especially if 4 tabs of Omega 3 (fish oil) tabs/d are ordered to lower triglycerides.

When I practiced Infectious Disease, I learned from HIV patients will take a huge number of pills to save their lives. Compliance was often determined with frequent HIV virus count.

I strongly believe the big problem with side-effect with statins is from starting at too high a dose.

Enduracin is over the counter at $90 for 1,000 tablets when purchased on the Internet. At the low dose it is unlikely the bad sides effects seen in AIM HIGH and HPS-THRIVE.

I started using this drug when other clinicians clued me into the fact this wax matrix preparation causes much less flush, especially if taken at breakfast or lunch. Most other Doctors advise taking at bedtime to deal with the hot flush that occurs. This probably wrong in that some authorities believe Niacin must be taken early in the day.

Zeta has finally had a positive outcome trial right at the time of the generic version (ezetimibe)becoming available.

If we truly want to prevent atherosclerotic heart disease we need to treat people earlier and for life to keep their LDLp under 750 or 1,000 or apo B around 60. This is the multiplier effect. A complex plaque that has been present for a long time will unlikely be cured with medications. However we need to treat early to prevent the simple plaque from becoming complex. Thus the legacy safety and price and efficacy call for the option of triple therapy before Injection PCSK9 which is very expensive and no legacy of safety or efficacy.

22

THE MULTIPLIER EFFECT

The Tubby Theory treats patients very early in their disease.

Even if the risk calculator was less than 10% over 10 years, I advised statin therapy if atherosclerosis was present on CAC or CIMT.

I believed any amount of plaque or atheroma was potentially deadly and it's progression should be stopped with a low LDLp < 1,000 or non-HDLc level <100.

I also advised getting the LDLp < 750 or non-HDLc level < 80 in order to get regression of plaque.

In 2010 this was aggressive approach.

In 2016 it has become much more acceptable.

Tuesday, June 28, 2016

Update on Multiplier effect with using statins early in treating CVD.

My theory called, The Multiplier effect, has been touted by me since I described using it in my lipidology practice in my 2009 book titled:

The Tubby Theory Theory from Topeka, published in 2010.

In a research letter on May 18, 2016 in JAMA. Dr. Sniderman writes:

"Our findings highlight the need to refine strategies to identify individuals younger than 60 years who are candidates for preventive therapies.

SEVERAL OPTIONS EXIST:

1. The risk threshold used by the lipid guidelines could be lowered to the optional 5% level,
2. or age and sex specific thresholds could be adopted,
3. additional risk factors might be added."

In 2009 in Topeka I was getting non-HDLc, LDLp, CAC and CIMT on my patients.

As with other models in treating chronic disease; hypertension, HIV, diabetes use multiple drugs for more efficacy and at lower doses to minimize the side effects for lifelong therapy.

The same is true to lower LDLp or apoB or non-HDLc.

In my medical practice before 2009 I was advising low dose simvastatin with 1,000 mg Endur-acin or Slo-niacin for less than $100 a year. If treatment goal not met, to then add Zetia.

In 2017 there is generic ezetimibe (Zetia), but not yet inexpensive. Generic atorvastatin (Lipitor) is available at very low price.

Generic rosuvastatin (Crestor) is also available and should be at a lower price.

The multiplier effect of combining these drugs and giving them early before complex plaque lesions occur hopefully will reduce the 30% residual risk considerably.

The new drug is PCSK9. Very expensive but the recent Fourier trial showed no serious side effects with LDLc of 30. The lower LDLc showed 15% less cardiovascular events in statin plus PCS9K arm vs. statin alone control arm.

This trial continues to validate that lower is better with LDLc.

REFERENCES

1. In obese, Insulin triggers steroidogenic factor (SF-1) which promotes food intake and perpetuates obesity. Vogt et. al. CNS Signaling Trends in Endo Metab 2013; 24(2) p76-84.

2. The action of Insulin on the Reward Pathway Dopaminergic is thought to contribute to development of obesity, since signaling of these higher neuronal circuits can override hypothalamic signaling.

   High sugar or high fat diet leads to neuronal insulin resistance and dysregulation of dopamine homeostasis and dopamine homeostasis leading to HYPODOPAMINERGIC REWARD DEFICIT SYNDROME.

   Wagner et al

3. *Marc-Andre Cornier et al*

   "Overexpression of FOXC2 has also been shown to prevent dietary induced obesity and insulin resistance in mice". Although the precise mechanisms of up-regulation of FOXC2 is unknown, its expression has been shown to be enhanced by insulin and an HF diet (27,28).

   With this in mind, we measured expression of adipose tissue **FOXC2** in a subset of participants (IS, *N* 8; IR, *N* 7) before and after the dietary intervention (27).

   Preliminary data suggest differential expression of FOXC2 in the IS and IR individuals in response to diets differing in macronutrient composition.

   In those two groups *who lost the most weight,* the dietary intervention resulted in substantial increases in FOXC2 expression, whereas in the two groups *with lesser weight loss,* FOXC2 expression remained unchanged."

   This is a small part of the hormonal regulation to cause weight regain in the reduced obese. The solution to maintain weight loss is with diet medications that correct these problems

4. Ebeling et al JAMA 2012; 307(24): 2627-2634

"Among overweight and obese young adults compared with pre-weight loss energy expenditure, isocaloric feeding following 10-15% weight loss resulted in decreases in REE and TEE that were greatest with:

1. the low fat diet,
2. intermediate with the low glycemic index diet and
3. least with the very low CHO diet.

5. A Novel Intervention Including Individualized Nutritional Recommendations Reduces Hemoglobin A1c Level, Medication Use, and Weight in Type 2 Diabetes

- Amy L McKenzie[1], PhD ;
- Sarah J Hallberg[1,2], DO, MS ;
- Published on 07.03.17 in **Vol 2, No 1 (2017): Jan-Jun**

Original Paper

"Conclusions: These initial results indicate that an individualized program delivered and supported remotely that incorporates nutritional ketosis can be highly effective in improving glycemic control and weight loss in adults with T2D while significantly decreasing medication use."

Most patients will have some ketones in their blood after fasting 12 hours. If they don't they may be resistant to doing well on an Atkins type diet and may explain some prior failures. It may also mean they need to fast the first and maybe second day when starting a diet. The nutritional ketosis fasting puts you in should help compliance with your diet. At least for the short term (6 to 9 months).

6. Frank Greenway recent review of Obesity Medicine :

International Journal of Obesity (2015) 39, 1188–1196; doi:10.1038/ijo.2015.59; published online 26 May 2015

"Following gastric bypass surgery, levels of ghrelin are extremely low, while GLP-1 and PYY are elevated, which should attenuate appetite."

7. <u>Ochner et al article Feb 11, 2015 link</u>

"Many clinicians are not adequately aware of the reasons that individuals with obesity struggle to achieve and maintain weight loss,[1] and this poor awareness precludes the provision of effective intervention.[2]

Excellent diet books

1. *The New Atkins for a New You* by Westman, Phinney and Votek 2010
2. *Always Hungry?* by David Ludwig MD, PhD
3. *Change Your Biology Diet* by Louis J. Aronne MD
4. *South Beach Diet* by Arthur Agatston MD
5. *The Diet Fix. Why diets fail and how to make yours work* by Yoni Freedhoff.
6. *New Hippocratic Diet guide* by Dr Irving A. Cohen
7. From a Prominent Death, Some Painful Truths

By <u>DENISE GRADY</u> **JUNE 24, 2008, NYT**

EPILOGUE

The main message of this book is that The Sponge Syndrome will cause weight gain despite Atkins because the low leptin levels tell your brain you are starving and it will use compensatory hormonal pathways to make a reduced obese patient gain weight.

I believe by my personal experience of having Chronic Obesity that the only way to maintain weight for greater than 10 years with satiety is with the addition of multiple diet medications.

Major challenges to treatment of chronic obesity:

1. Diet Medication high cost
2. Must stay on diet medication for rest of life.
3. Must stay on restrictive diet for rest of life.

People are offered bariatric surgery rather than trying a LCHF diet with nutritional ketosis.

Physicians must learn about diet medications and use them as a first drug, especially if on Insulin, rather than the last medication to try.

Don't ever tell a reduced obese patient, they regained weight because they didn't exercise enough (60 to 90 minutes/day) or stick to a starvation diet (1500 cal/day and one hour of exercise) despite this being the present guideline to maintain weight loss.

Ask your Doctor if he had read Gina Kolata NYT article on *The Biggest Loser*. They regained even though they did everything right.

It is all about never losing your fat cells. When adipocytes are shrunken in the reduced obese, they are low in Leptin and tell your brain you are starving and MiRNA from the numerous fat cells bring the same message to most of the body in the form of episomes. Remember 70% of your resting metabolism is from the liver, brain and kidney. When these organs are tuned down in metabolism no amount of exercise can overcome it. More exercise makes a patient more hungry in patients with the disease of chronic obesity.

The only way to fight this is with diet medications.

Finally find a physician certified in the American Board of Obesity Medicine who has a good bioelectric impedance weight scale so you can follow your muscle mass. It will be discouraging to see the 5-10% loss of muscle mass as you lose weight. I think it is more important to lose as much weight as possible in the 6 to 9 month window. Then at the plateau, start the low weight high repetition (24 reps, 3 sets, 4 times a week) exercises on very high protein diet (2.4 mg/d protein per kg of lean body weight).

With more exercise is more hunger. This is why you will need the diet medications more than ever.

I had 44.2 lbs of muscle by bioelectric impedance scale on 11-6-15 with 235.1 lbs of weight.

I started to go to Stormont Obesity Clinic run by Dr. Jennifer Scheid (Board Certified in Obesity Medicine) on 6-23-15. After a month of weight lifting and water aerobics, I weighed 244.8 lbs with **46.1 lbs of muscle mass.**

After diet medications and continuing Atkins type diet and walking only 1-2 miles a day I came home from a Wedding weekend in Philadelphia and a National Lipid Association meeting on 5-23-17, and weighed 199 lbs with 37.4 lbs of muscle mass.

My present goal is to do 24 reps of low weights a day alternating legs and upper body with more effort to gaining weight in the leg muscles. I will also try to eat 2.4 g of protein/kg of lean body weight.

Lean body weight at 199 lbs is 150 lbs.

My visceral fat is 13.

I hope to reach the goal of visceral fat of 9 or less with more muscle mass. It is more important than the actual total lbs of weight.

I will report my future efforts on my blog. (http://meandgin.blogspot.com/)

SUMMARY

The multiple diet medicines have helped me maintain my weight loss from 280 lbs to 200 lbs from Feb 2006 till _11 years later_.

I think Atkins was essential as I ate ad libitum and *was never hungry*. I didn't really lose weight on Atkins, I mostly stopped gaining weight even though I decreased my exercise from 2 hours a day to walking 20-40 minutes a day. I lost significant weight when I added the diet medications Jan 1, 2018 weight 204.2 pounds

GLOSSARY

THE BLOOD TESTS

1. **LDL-C**: the C stands for cholesterol. This is the bad cholesterol. It is determined from a blood test. It is a calculated number and is often discordant with the newer better test, LDL-P. The P stands for particle.

2. **LDL-P:** The number of particles (P) that carry the cholesterol, is the best predictor of cardiovascular risk. It is determined by a blood test and an NMR machine. ApoB is another way to measure the atherogenic particles. High fat diets make large LDL-P, while low fat diets make for more small dense LDL-P. There is much confusion about size being important for risk stratification. The National Lipid Association meetings preach that size doesn't matter most of the time. No double entendre intended.

3. **HDL-C:** This has been called the good cholesterol. Ratios are often used to determine cardiovascular risk. The AIM-HIGH trial and the fact that there are pro-inflammatory or bad HDL-C's makes the ratio with HDL-C less reliable. Low fat diets lower HDL-C. High fat diets raise HDL-C.

4. **HDL-P**: The particle number will raise with the HDL-C till about a level of 60 dl/ml. At this point as the HDL-C goes higher, the size of the HDL-P gets larger. What does it all mean? It's a conundrum as the critical test is the functionality of the HDL-P. There is no clinical lab test for functionality at this time.

5. **Triglycerides:** 3 fatty acids make up a triglyceride. Low carbohydrate diets have low triglycerides. Low fat diets have high triglycerides.

6. **Tubby Factor:** I coined this term as the technical term *non-HDL Cholesterol* was too confusing. This is the second best predictor of cardiovascular risk. It is all the cholesterol without the HDL-C. Take the Total Cholesterol level on your lipid panel and subtract the HDL-C. This is also often discordant with the LDL-C especially in people with metabolic syndrome.

MEDICAL IMAGING:

7. **CAC (coronary calcium score):** This is a CT scan of the heart. It can show if a patient has plaque in his coronary arteries. No IV, no dye involved.

8. **CIMT (carotid intima medial wall thickness):** ultrasound of the carotid arteries in the neck that measures the thickness of the wall of the carotid. It is different from the duplex carotid ultrasound that measures the flow of the blood in the carotid and determines how much blockage there is in the carotid.

DIABETIC TERMS:

9. **Metabolic syndrome:** This is a prediabetic state with apple obesity, high blood pressure, high triglycerides and low HDL-C.
10. **Hgb A1C:** Hemoglobin A1C is a blood test to determine the average glucose level in the blood over the last one or two months.
11. **Prediabetes:** a fasting glucose 100 or greater.
12. **Apple obesity:** a waist greater than 40 inches in male or 35 inches in a female.
13. **High Blood Pressure:** greater than 130 systolic
14. **High Triglycerides:** greater than 150
15. **Low HDL-C:** lower than 40 for males and lower than 50 for females

Reduced obese: a person who has lost a significant amount of weight and now has a different metabolism from obese people and normal weight people. The reduced obese now has a body that is using several compensatory mechanisms to gain weight.

SET POINT:

"Metab Syndr Relat Disord. 2011 Apr;9(2):85-9. Epub 2010 Nov 30.
Set-point theory and obesity.
Farias MM, Cuevas AM, Rodriguez F.
Source
Department of Nutrition and Metabolism, Pontificia Universidad Catolica de Chile, Santiago, Chile.

Abstract
Obesity is a consequence of the complex interplay between genetics and environment. Several studies have shown that body weight is maintained at a stable range, known as the "set-point," despite the variability in energy intake and expenditure. Additionally, it has been shown that the body is more efficient protecting against weight loss during caloric deprivation compared to conditions of weight gain with overfeeding, suggesting an adaptive role of protection during periods of low food intake. Emerging evidence on bariatric surgery outcomes, particularly gastric bypass, suggests a novel role of these surgical procedures in establishing a new set-point by alterations in body weight regulatory physiology, therefore resulting in sustainable weight loss results. Continuing research is necessary to elucidate the

biological mechanisms responsible for this change, which may offer new options for the global burden of obesity."

Plateau: After 8% or more weight loss, it becomes difficult to lose more weight.

Re-settlement point: New term for plateau? Obese people have high levels of leptin. Some believe this is a resistance as with insulin. Others believe the obesse have a high leptin threshold. Fat cells make leptin. As the fat cells shrink, less leptin is made. If the threshold is high in the obese, and the leptin level goes below a threshold which alerts the brain that the body is starving, the body starts compensatory mechanisms to gain the weight back.

Energy gap: "These formulas would predict an energy gap of 190-200 kcal/day for a 100 kg person losing 10% of body weight and an energy gap of 280-300 kcal/day for this same person losing 15% of body weight (Figure 4). The energy gap for weight loss maintenance can provide an estimate of how much behavior change is required to maintain a given amount of weight loss. This analysis indicates that in order to create and maintain significant body weight loss (i.e. obesity treatment) large behavioral changes are needed. This is in stark contrast to primary obesity prevention in which small behavioral changes can eliminate the small energy imbalance that occurs before the body has gained significant weight. Because the body has not previously stored this "new" excess energy, it does not defend against the behavioral strategies as happens when the body loses weight."

J Am Diet Assoc. Author manuscript; available in PMC 2010 November 1.

Published in final edited form as:

J Am Diet Assoc. 2009 November; 109(11): 1848–1853.

doi: 10.1016/j.jada.2009.08.007

PMCID: PMC2796109

NIHMSID: NIHMS155611

Copyright notice and Disclaimer

Using the Energy Gap to Address Obesity: A Commentary

James O. Hill, Ph.D., Professor of Pediatrics and Medicine, Director,John C. Peters, Ph.D., Associate Director, and Holly R. Wyatt, M.D., Associate Professor

Leptin threshold: "Dieting means less fat in your body's fat cells, and it also means a lower level of leptin. When you go below your personal leptin threshold, your brain thinks you're starving. The body has ways of handling this apparent crisis, initiating a number of processes designed to keep you from starving, and raise the level of leptin back up above your personal leptin threshold. Unfortunately these processes can also sabotage your diet." Jody Smith June 2010.

Leptin resistance: "Although leptin is a circulating signal that reduces appetite, obese individuals generally exhibit an unusually high circulating concentration of leptin. [56] These people are said to be resistant to the effects of leptin, in much the same way that people with type 2 diabetes are resistant to the effects of insulin. The high sustained concentrations of leptin from the enlarged adipose stores result in leptin desensitization. The pathway of leptin control in obese people might be flawed at some point so the body does not adequately receive the satiety feeling subsequent to eating." From Wikipedia

Sponge Syndrome: I coined this term because the definitions above are very complicated and not yet fully understood. I know from personal experience that after losing 80 pounds, I gained 58 pounds despite 2-3 hours of exercise a day over a 43 month period. I gained 1.35 pounds a month. I gained weigh like a sponge due to my body's energy gap that develops after losing weight and this energy gap gets larger as the amount of weight loss gets larger.

Moral hazard of obesity: Once someone is obese there is a general belief that weight loss should only be obtained through deprivation and exercise. If someone is fat, it is their own fault.

The theory that weight loss can be maintained with a high fat diet and little exercise is impossible.

National Weight Control Registry found people who maintained weight loss did aspects of success. Many guidelines base their recommendations on this.

1. weigh themselves every day and then if 3-5 pounds heavier, they had a *plan* what to do about it immediately
2. they tended to have little variety in their food
3. they splurged less on food on holidays.
4. they ate *1,385 calories/day* but the facilitator said they are under reporting
5. they ate 4.87 meals a day
6. they linked behaviors to something more than just losing weight.

For example they use walking as their social time. They linked good behaviors to something they want to do.

7. they often had a life changing event such as divorce or new job.
8. they walk about five miles a day or exercise equivalent

It's also reported in Medical Clinics of North America Sept 2011 V 95 #5
on page 945:
"The National Weight Control 'Registry documented the metabolic and behavioral cost of maintaining a weight loss for more than 5 years. The average weight loss was 30 kg (66 lbs) and minimum maintenance 13.6 kg. (29.92 lbs.) The results are instructive. Both men and women consumed low-fat diet (24%) and exercised to use 470 and 360 kcal/d, respectively. The net energy balance was 918 kcal/day for women and 1225 kcal/d for men. These reduced obese ate an average of five meals a day and conducted a very regimented existence."

ANCEL KEYS GREAT STARVATION EXPERIMENT:

Compare this World War Two experiment to the NWCR the 8 items listed above.

Thirty two volunteers were feed approximately 1550/cal a day for six months.

The subjects walked 3 miles a day.

The subject suffered mentally and physically. A few of them were caught eating garbage when they didn't lose weight and were kicked out of the experiment.

This is the same diet most guidelines tell patients to adhere to presently.

This is insanity. The good news is that there is medicine to prevent the severe hunger. The bad news is most Doctors and patients don't know about or don't want to take a diet medicine for the rest of their lives.

Printed in the United States
By Bookmasters